T0129164

Cancer
MADE ME
Beautiful

Cancer
MADE ME
Beautiful

Cherie A. Hunter

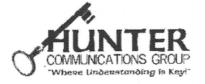

HUNTER
COMMUNICATIONS GROUP
"Where Understanding is Key!"

AuthorHouse™
1663 Liberty Drive
Bloomington, IN 47403
www.authorhouse.com
Phone: 1-800-839-8640

This publication contains the opinions and ideas of its author. It is intended to provide helpful and informative material on the subject matter covered. It is sold with the understanding that the publisher is not engaged in rendering psychological, medical, or other professional services. If expert assistance or counseling is needed, the services of a competent professional should be sought.

First published by AuthorHouse   05/26/2011

ISBN: 978-1-4634-1062-9 (sc)
ISBN: 978-1-4634-1061-2 (ebk)

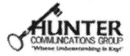

www.huntercommunicationsinc.com
Cover design by Erial Ramsey, Design Diva

Printed in the United States of America

Reviews

"Cherie shows us how to actively participate in our health care and how important it is for the family and the village to participate in every step of the journey to Recovery"

Funeka Sihlali, MJ, R.N.

"This book is a "must-read" not only for persons living with cancer; but also for their family members, their significant others and for persons who are wrestling with "unseen [and unnamed] forces. I guarantee you; Cancer Made Me Beautiful's clarity will be life changing for you."

Reverend Dr. Jeremiah A. Wright, Jr.,
Pastor Emeritus Trinity United Church of Christ

"How wonderful the title, Cancer Made Me Beautiful: A Journey to Recovery. Cherie Hunter has taken her experience with an illness that many view as ugly and turned it into a recovery journey that readers will no doubt view as beautiful. When I read her story I was amazed by the similarities in our experiences. She is recovering from cancer and I am in recovery from a 13 year addiction to heroin. When I read her book it felt as if she were telling my recovery story. I am convinced whatever your ailment, disease or disorder, whether it is cancer, drug addiction, or trauma, you will want to read this book. It will provide you with a pathway to recovery that clearly reveals the power of God in each of us. Sit back and relax as the author leads you on a journey to recovery!"

David Njabulo Whiters, PhD
ClarkAtlanta University
Adjunct Professor
Person in long-term addiction recovery

Reviews (continued)

"If there is one book that has the potential to really define and teach how to recover from a seemingly hopeless life experience, this is it. I believe that Cherie, using her own experience with Cancer, will change the way we look at this disease. The stigma and fear of this disease will become myths and the 'fact of the truth' reality."
Lonnetta Albright, Executive Director,
Great Lakes Addiction Technology Transfer Center

"Cancer Made Me Beautiful" is a personal revelation about becoming the best we want ourselves to be. Cherie's struggle and the management of her cancer helped reveal to herself the innate strength and beauty she possessed. It is the story of a personal awakening. It is also the story of a remarkable family whose, love, commitment and spiritual energy produce generations of beautiful people."
Melody M. Heaps, President Emeritus,
Treatment Alternatives for Safe Communities (TASC)

"That, which does not kill you will only make you stronger, is a lesson learned and then taught by this book. So I say to the reader, beware. If self-pity and defeat is where you find your comfort zone, Cancer Made Me Beautiful will surely be what frustrates you to a point of crossroad."
Minister Lonnie V. Hunter III, Brother

In Loving Memory of:
MY FATHER, LONNIE HUNTER (1919 – 2011)

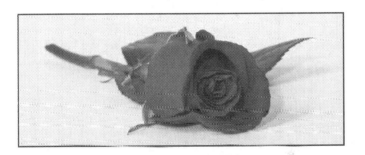

Dedications

In loving memory of my mother Augusta Dooley Hunter who lost her battle to colon cancer in 1973, but gave me all she had in the short period I had her in my life. By your example you gave me Grace, Wisdom, Patience, and Perseverance, but most of all you gave me Jesus.

In memory of my sister/friend Vernola Baskin, who lost her battle to lung cancer in 2008. You showed me how to have grace even in death. I love you my sister.

To all of our loved ones who fought a good fight and all of the survivors who continue to inspire, encourage and role model perseverance in the battle with the enemy we call cancer.

Acknowledgements

With my appreciation and love, I would like to thank my family for their love and support during my illness, recovery and the writing of this book. Without you this book would not have been possible. I thank God daily for allowing me to be born into such a loving and caring family.

A special thanks and much love goes out to my sister Lonnetta Albright who has always believed in me and my ability to write this book, even when I didn't believe in myself.

With thanksgiving and gratitude, I thank Pastor Emeritus, Rev. Dr. Jeremiah A. Wright and the entire ministerial staff of Trinity United Church of Christ. You helped me to reconcile my past with my faith and through your teaching, gave me back my life by helping me connect to my spirit within.

Finally, I want to extend my thanks to the management and staff of Treatment Alternatives for Safe Communities (TASC), who as my employer and colleagues became my extended family for support, comfort and encouragement. I love you all.

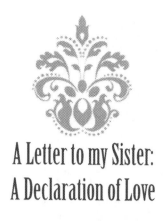

A Letter to my Sister: A Declaration of Love

LONNIE V. HUNTER III

Dear Cherie,

I am a firm believer that the trials and tribulations we face are never solely for our own benefit. We face challenges (however great or small) to become equipped with a unique testimony that will serve as reassurance to those that come after us, that God is still able. You are a shining example of what it means to turn lemons into lemonade.

Throughout this whole process, from diagnosis to complete healing, I have watched you go to battle through emotional and physical valleys and consistently come out a winner. To say that I am proud of you would be an understatement.

Your account of the battle you faced brought things to the forefront that I never even knew you were going through. Your grace, determination, spiritual connection, and die hard attitude are clearly what have qualified you to write a book of this caliber. As the pages turn, you have an ability to write so visually that any reader, going through any type of setback, can pull wisdom and strength; giving the reader a new more positive attitude on life and the ups and downs it has to offer. I salute you in seeing the need and having the compassion not to hold back on your story. You, being the type of quality woman of God you are, have seen this storm as a way to build the Kingdom and lessen the effects the enemy has attached to such a diagnosis.

That, which does not kill you will only make you stronger, is a lesson learned and then taught by this book. So I say to the reader, beware. If self-pity and defeat are where you find your comfort zone, the pages to come will surely be what frustrate you to a point of crossroad. Will my situation kill me? Or will it make me stronger?

Cherie, what makes you great in my eyes, is your desire to not only recognize greatness in yourself, but to help others recognize the greatness within them.

If I haven't told you lately, I love you. You are my she-ro. You honor me and my work by joining me as I release my newest CD. Who knew as I wrote the words to "I'm Back" that they would speak to your heart and life as they did mine.

So Cherie once again we soar together, we journey together and we both know that God is the center of our joy and the source of our strength. As insufficient as the phrase is, it is nonetheless true.... I AM PROUD OF YOU!!

I Love You,
Lonnie

Table of Contents

Preface:
A Balm of Honesty

REVEREND DR. JEREMIAH A. WRIGHT, JR.

The expression "brutally honest" always carries a negative connotation with it. Cherie Hunter, however, has an honesty in this book that is not "brutal." Cherie's honesty is a balm that will heal many believers deep down in their spirits! When Cherie says, "I found myself unable to reconcile my faith with what was going on in my reality," she puts her finger on the pulse of the pain which throbs in the souls of millions of believers who struggle with that same issue.

Her honesty opens up the hidden wound, the unmentionable misery and the masked malaise that keep many people of faith from being able to begin the healing process. Her honesty not only debrides that wound, however, Cherie's honesty allows the fresh air of God's grace to get inside the hurt where the "wrestling" takes place; and it applies the Balm in Gilead to the source of the pain, breaking the silence and starting the healing process in an exciting, surprising and transformative way.

When the reader comes to grips with the raw truth and honesty Cherie exudes on the pages of *Cancer Made Me Beautiful*, and when the reader realizes that one of their unnamed issues is that they too have been unable to "reconcile [their] faith with what is going on in [their] reality," the Balm of Grace and God's healing will begin its work in their souls; and they will experience what the Apostle Paul writes about when he says that God has begun a work in them and that God will continue that work until it is brought to completion.

Cherie's honesty will open the eyes, the minds and the hearts of any reader who earnestly seeks an answer to life's most difficult questions. This book is a "must-read" not only for persons living with cancer; but also for their family members and their significant others.

It is also a "must-read" for persons who are wrestling with "unseen [and unnamed] forces" as Jacob wrestled by the River Jabbok. I guarantee you; *Cancer Made Me Beautiful*'s clarity will be life-changing for you.

Reverend Dr. Jeremiah A. Wright, Jr.
Pastor Emeritus
Trinity United Church of Christ
Chicago, Illinois
March 2011

Foreword

MONICA MOSS

You have cancer. I can clearly remember every circumstance surrounding the moment that my life was forever changed by those three small, yet powerful words. You have cancer. There had to be some mistake. I had no family history, I didn't smoke, I ate a healthy diet and exercised. I was a person of Faith. I was a Pastor's wife for goodness sake! I was a new mother with two small children who needed me to be there for them to help them to grow and to become. I had no time to be sick, let alone deal with the disruption of cancer.

However, the reality is that the vast majority of us will someday be confronted, whether directly or indirectly, with the actuality of cancer. If we are not the recipient of the diagnosis, more than likely a close relative, friend or loved one will experience this dreaded disease. Yet, there is hope and a cancer diagnosis is not a guaranteed death sentence.

A diagnosis is just that – a diagnosis. The way in which we deal with the diagnosis is what empowers us to endure the battle or to be defeated. In *Cancer Made Me Beautiful*, Cherie Hunter gives us a first-hand account of her journey through her battle with cancer as well as the life-affirming lessons she learned in the process. Her courageous story gives us hope to know that the greatest challenges of our lives possess the most meaningful lessons for our own personal transformation.

Cancer Made Me Beautiful is an empowering story of fortitude that will help the person experiencing the ramifications of cancer as well as anyone who finds him or herself in a battle for courage, self-realization or perseverance. By generously offering the candid and moving accounts of her own healing journey as an example of triumph and victory over the giant of cancer in her life, Cherie has gifted us with a tool for overcoming obstacles and becoming more powerful. She has given us a roadmap for creating an environment for healing filled with abundance, balance, love and peace.

This book is important because it demonstrates that there is no challenge, including cancer or illness, greater than the power we possess as children of God. Our faith is what strengthens us and allows us to realize that with Christ we are more than conquerors in all things and in all ways. Allow this book, this testimony, to assist you on your own journey to wholeness and a full and fruitful life. Take these life lessons and tools for action and healing to heart. *Cancer Made Me Beautiful* will help you to understand how your feelings and emotions impact your wellbeing as well as how we can be released from those things that truly hinder our freedom of spirit, creativity and joy even as we face the greatest adversities of our lives.

God be with you,
Monica Moss

Romans 12:1-2...Be transformed by the renewing of your mind.

Introduction

LONNETTA M. ALBRIGHT

"In all your ways acknowledge him, and he will make straight your paths"
Proverbs 3:6, NRSV

Cancer Made Me Beautiful and its author have found a way to take a scary and serious circumstance; and turn it into something courageous, soft and inspiring. If there is one book that has the potential to really define and teach how to recover from a seemingly hopeless life experience, this is it. I believe that Cherie, using her own experience with Cancer, will change the way we look at this disease. The stigma and fear of this disease will become myths and the "fact of the truth" reality.

The words Cancer and Beauty are strongly marked opposites. To achieve a balance of opposites is a daunting task. An idealist is not usually realistic, a fearful person is not usually courageous, a pragmatist is not a risk taker, nor a risk taker a pragmatic. "But life at its best is a creative synthesis of opposites in fruitful harmony" (Strength to Love, Martin Luther King). Cherie has mastered this harmony in her first book that not only achieves a creative synthesis but also blends the head and heart of the matter.

When sharing her vision for the title of this book many would look at her a little strangely and ask, how does cancer and beauty live in the same place? What about cancer suggest anything that exemplifies beauty? Isn't this disease awful and dark and hopeless; so how does this beauty piece fit?

The answers to these questions are found in this uniquely crafted book that blends facts with real life; spirituality with physiology; education with personal experiences and fear with victory. As a matter of fact, in the pages that follow there are many answers.

The book is written in a way that offers revelations and truths that the author learned along her journey -- answers about cancer; answers about what it takes to recover and answers that offer hope, encouraging the reader to find their own divine power to take control of their own recovery and ultimately their own lives. "We are in control" -- that is the essence of this book. Recovery and Transformation are the outcomes.

The book has a rhythm that dramatically crescendos. It uses the beat of the author's heart, the thoughts and reflections of her mind, her quick wit and self-effacing humor to tell her personal story. A story that weaves repeatedly and consistently a number of themes throughout: setting the context – educating along the way – deep and abiding spirituality – a lived experience

– support of loved ones and the community – lessons learned – a recovery and transformation process.

In Chapter 1 – *Unraveling the Mystery,* we begin to understand one of the author's personal beliefs and values – 'knowledge is power'. And that power, personal power; is what is needed to overcome any challenge. In this opening chapter the author begins the education process at the highest level. She walks us through a detailed understanding of cancer in a way that we can and should understand. Her inquiring mind; coupled with research, study and prayer are tools that serve well enough in conveying the "truth of the matter" in an attempt to unravel and debunk the power of the unknown. First taking the time to educate, the reader will more accurately understand the language that follows throughout the book and hopefully begin to dispel the usual fear and stigma related to the "Big C".

In Chapter 2 – *Exposing the Enemy,* the story begins to unfold and we start to see how faith, education, family support and courage are needed when faced with confusing and traumatic experiences. Using a chronology of events, Cherie carefully draws us into her head and heart. We can feel her emotions; understand her deliberate and inquisitive search for understanding; and her unswerving faith and courage. Courage that surprised her at times and yet when all was said and done, confirmed that we can take control of our own lives.

In Chapter 3, *The Dance,* Cherie begins to achieve the "balance of opposites". Anger and joy undergird this chapter. She moves between the past and present, back and forth through her life. Looking back she comes face to face with what she feared most, repeating her mother's unsuccessful battle with cancer; and what she loves most – family. The questions, revelations, anger (with God) and reconciliation with her past help to propel her forward. It is in this chapter where we learn how important education, family and faith helped to build her courage, fortitude and hope.

Chapter 4, *Wholeness: Recovery on all Levels* marks the turning point. The rhythm is building. So much energy and excitement are felt in these pages. Blending what's known in her field of work as "recovery capital" we see the value of the people in her life, the strength of her faith, her tireless quest for knowledge and understanding and her sheer gratitude for the experience. She also carefully sheds some light on addiction – her early addiction to the pain medication associated with the treatment of this disease. She comes to know herself more fully and believes that acceptance of who we are brings about forgiveness, transformation and genuine recovery. She calls this 'the new normal".

Chapter 5, *Hitting the Reset Button* – This is my favorite chapter, likely due to the fact that I am an educator and enjoy sharing information with others. But not just any type of education. I believe, as does Cherie, that in learning there has to be reconciliation, if you will; of heart and head. This chapter achieves that balance. On the one hand Cherie presents a process that she has titled "Hitting the Reset Button: Bringing Balance Back into Your Life". But here again, she first educates us and puts the process in context building upon her own experiences, lessons learned and guided always by her faith in God. Capitalizing upon her 12-month journey she introduces a process and steps that again balances opposites --challenges as opportunities.

Chapter 6, *Transformation* is the final chapter. At the start of the chapter her scripture reference, "So if anyone be in Christ, he is a new creation: everything old has passed away; behold, everything has become new!" (2 Corinthians 5:17 NRSV) sets the stage for the remaining pages. We see her courage. We see her joy. We see her new normal. She travels to Africa, accomplishes the "Deacon Walk" at her church, is now speaking to and performing in front of audiences (previously she'd always chosen to be in the background), she's excelling in her professional life and her personal announcement is "I'm Back". And as only she can do, her life is intimately connected to her family. There is no coincidence and certainly no accident that her brother's newest Gospel CD single, "I'm Back" touched her heart. And again there's the rhythm.

While I had the privilege and honor to personally watch and be involved in Cherie's story, I am still blown away with the elegance, depth of emotion, talent, devotion to God, family and all people that makes her the woman that she is--the author that she's become. Cherie's beauty and the beauty of this book simultaneously speaks to a broad range of readers; from survivors to those currently battling the Big C, family members, loved ones, caretakers and professionals. She rallies us all to educate ourselves, support each other and take back our personal power. And even though she believes this to be her first and only book I suspect that we will hear from her again and again.

CHAPTER ONE

Unraveling the Mystery

"For my thoughts are not your thoughts, neither are your ways my ways," declares the LORD.
Isaiah 55:8

The diagnosis is Lymphoma Cancer. These were the words spoken to me in June, 2005 that changed the trajectory of my life forever. They were the very words I feared most, so naturally they shook me to my core. I was about to begin a journey with an unknown outcome, not to mention hidden twists and turns. Every part of my being, and who I thought I was; was about to be tested. And I didn't know if I had what it took to pass the examination. Over the next year I would experience an increase in my love of family, belief in self and my level of faith. Life as I once knew it would be no more.

The critical questions that had to be answered were; what was lymphoma and why was it attacking me? I knew the enemy called Cancer hovered over us all, lying in wait to devour who and what it could. But this particular form of cancer called lymphoma, I knew nothing about. Where did it come from? What was its cause? And most of all, what had I done that permitted it to enter my life? It was all a mystery; requiring research, study and prayer in an attempt to unravel and debunk its power.

This book has been in the making for the last five years. While finally putting pen to paper (Nov 2010), I am celebrating my 5th anniversary of completion of treatment, placing me officially on the remission list. But in looking back over the experience, as well as sitting by the bedside of others stricken by the disease of cancer, I realize that there are some feelings that we all experience at one point or another – Depression, Anger, Fear and Hopelessness.

It was difficult for me to accept my calling to write such a book or to move forward with the process of writing. After all, I was just an everyday woman who had given her life to Christ and allowed God to heal and deliver her. I did not have a major platform, nor was I in the public eye. So who would listen to me? Nevertheless, my hesitancy and apprehension did not matter to God. Though the writing process was slow and long in coming; I had to take a deep breath, say my prayers and finally, literally, be pushed into this process.

I recognize that people with cancer, no matter the type, faced the same obstacles as anyone else striving for recovery. I believe that while we attempt to separate recovery into categories; such as weight loss, alcohol, drugs or illness, the steps taken to achieve full recovery are the same. Since my experience or road to recovery came through Cancer, I knew it would have to be the recovery platform from which I had to speak.

In this, my first book; I not only give you a glimpse into the journey of a cancer survivor, but my intent is to also lay out a detailed and practical plan for bringing balance back into your life and restoring you to your purpose. In *Cancer Made Me Beautiful* I deal directly and powerfully with the spiritual and psychological barriers that stand in the way of our recovery on all levels when confronted with the harsh realities of life.

Throughout this book, I offer sensible, usable and even enjoyable steps you can use to overcome your fears, anxiety and other negative emotions; transforming them into life-affirming behaviors. No longer will you see your life in fragments. You will begin to see the whole picture that will allow you to live in your own power and restore your life's balance.

The Big C

The human face of cancer sometimes gets lost in the blizzard of statistics, stereotypes, and hyped-up media images. However, the disease of cancer touches almost every family in this day and age, while leaving many recipients of the disease and their families asking why or wondering what to do.

Now, cancer itself when defined in general terms by the American Cancer Society, is a class of diseases in which a cell, or a group of cells display uncontrolled growth (division beyond the normal limits), invasion (intrusion on and destruction of adjacent tissues), and sometimes metastasis (spread to other locations in the body via lymph or blood). These three malignant properties of cancers differentiate them from benign tumors, which are self-limited, and do not invade or metastasize. Most cancers form a tumor but some, like leukemia, do not. The area or specialty of medicine concerned with the study, diagnosis, treatment, and prevention of cancer is oncology.

Cancer can affect people at all ages with the risk for most types increasing with age. It caused about 13% of all human deaths in 2007 (7.6 million). Cancers are primarily an environmental disease with 90-95% of cases due to lifestyle and environmental factors and 5-10% due to genetics. Common environmental factors leading to cancer death include: tobacco (25-30%), diet and obesity (30-35%), infections (15-20%), radiation, stress, lack of physical activity and environmental pollutants. These environmental factors cause abnormalities in the genetic material of cells.

Genetic abnormalities found in cancer typically affect two general classes of genes. Cancer-promoting oncogenes are typically activated in cancer cells, giving those cells new properties, such as hyperactive growth and division, protection against programmed cell death, loss of respect for normal tissue boundaries, and the ability to become established in diverse tissue environments. Tumor suppressor genes are then inactivated in cancer cells, resulting in the loss of normal functions in those cells, such as accurate DNA replication, control over the cell cycle, orientation and adhesion within tissues, and interaction with protective cells of the immune system.

(Source: Wikipedia Foundation, Inc. www.wikipedia.org/wiki/AmericanCancerSociety, 2010)

Lymphoma as a Type

When I was diagnosed with Non-Hodgkin's Lymphoma during the summer of 2005, I had no idea what lymphoma was. I realized that if I didn't, there had to be many others lacking that same knowledge. So I set out to find out all I could about the disease. What I discovered was that lymphoma is a type of cancer involving cells of the immune system, called lymphocytes. Just as cancer represents many different diseases, lymphoma represents many different cancers of lymphocytes -- about 35 different subtypes, in fact.

So what does all of this mean? In the next few pages I offer a fairly detailed description and education on lymphoma as a type of cancer. Hopefully this information will help others facing this particular type of cancer.

Lymphoma is a group of cancers that affect the cells that play a role in the immune system and primarily represents cells involved in the lymphatic system of the body. The lymphatic system is part of the immune system. It consists of a network of vessels that carry fluid called lymph, similar to the way that the network of blood vessels carries blood throughout the body. Lymph contains white blood cells called lymphocytes. Lymphocytes attack a variety of infectious agents as well as many cells in the precancerous stages of development.

Lymph nodes are small collections of lymph tissue that occur throughout the body. The lymphatic system involves lymphatic channels that connect thousands of lymph nodes scattered throughout the body. Lymph flows through the lymph nodes, as well as through other lymphatic tissues including the spleen, the tonsils, the bone marrow, and the thymus gland.

These lymph nodes filter the lymph, which may carry bacteria, viruses, or other microbes. The lymph nodes, or glands as they may be called, filter the lymph; which may on various occasions carry different microbial organisms. At infection sites, large numbers of these microbial organisms collect in the regional lymph nodes and produce the swelling and tenderness typical of a localized infection. These enlarged and occasionally confluent collections of lymph nodes (so-called lymphadenopathy) are often referred to as "swollen glands." In some areas of the body (such as the anterior part of the neck), they are often visible when swollen.

Lymphocytes recognize infectious organisms and abnormal cells and destroy them. There are two major subtypes of lymphocytes: B lymphocytes and T lymphocytes also referred to as B cells and T cells.

B lymphocytes produce antibodies (proteins that circulate through the blood and lymph and attach to infectious organisms and abnormal cells). Antibodies essentially alert other cells of the immune system to recognize and destroy these intruders, also known as pathogens.

T cells, when activated, can kill pathogens directly. T cells also play a part in the mechanisms of immune system control, to prevent the system from inappropriate over-activity or under-activity. After fighting off an invader, some of the B and T lymphocytes remember the invader and are prepared to fight it off if it returns.

Cancer occurs when normal cells undergo a transformation whereby they grow and multiply uncontrollably. Lymphoma is a malignant transformation of either B or T cells or their subtypes. As the abnormal cells multiply, they may collect in one or more lymph nodes or in other lymph tissues such as the spleen. As the cells continue to multiply, they form a mass often referred to as a tumor. Tumors often overwhelm surrounding tissues by invading their space, thereby depriving them of the necessary oxygen and nutrients needed to survive and function normally.

In lymphoma, abnormal lymphocytes travel from one lymph node to the next, and sometimes to remote organs, via the lymphatic system. While lymphomas are often confined to lymph nodes and other lymphatic tissue, they can spread to other types of tissue almost anywhere in the body. Lymphoma development outside of lymphatic tissue is called extra-nodal disease.

Lymphomas fall into one of two major categories: Hodgkin's lymphoma (HL, previously called Hodgkin's disease) and all other lymphomas (non-Hodgkin's lymphomas or NHLs). I was diagnosed with the latter.

These two types occur in the same places, may be associated with the same symptoms, and often have similar appearance on physical examination. However, they are readily distinguishable via microscopic examination.

Hodgkin's disease develops from a specific abnormal B lymphocyte lineage. NHL may derive from either abnormal B or T cells and are distinguished by unique genetic markers. There are five subtypes of Hodgkin's disease and about 30 subtypes of non-Hodgkin's lymphoma.

Because there are so many different subtypes of lymphoma, the classification of lymphomas are complicated (it includes both the microscopic appearance as well as genetic and molecular markers). Many of the NHL subtypes look similar, but they are functionally quite different and respond to different therapies with different probabilities of cure. HL subtypes are microscopically distinct, and typing is based upon the microscopic differences as well as extent of disease.

Lymphoma is the most common type of blood cancer in the United States. It is the seventh most common cancer in adults and the third most common in children. Non-Hodgkin's lymphoma is far more common than Hodgkin's lymphoma.

In the United States, about 66,000 new cases of NHL and 8,500 new cases of HL were expected to be diagnosed in 2010, and the overall incidence is increasing each year. About 19,500 deaths due to NHL were expected in 2010 as well as 1,290 deaths due to HL, with the survival rate of all but the most advanced cases of HL greater than that of other lymphomas.

Lymphoma can occur at any age, including childhood. Hodgkin's disease is most common in two age groups: young adults 16-34 years of age and in older people 55 years of age and older. Non-Hodgkin's lymphoma is more likely to occur in older people.

(Source: Wikipedia Foundation, Inc. www.wikipedia.org/wiki/Lymphoma, 2011)

As I stated earlier, I was diagnosed with NHL, but I didn't fall in either of the most common age groups cited. But I have always been told that I was unique.

The probability of developing cancer in your lifetime in the United States is 44% for men and 38% for women. More and more people are being diagnosed with all types of cancer than ever before. In many ways, it's true that we are better off today than generations before us thanks to research, early diagnosis and treatment. Yet, in spite of all our advances in research, we still face fear, depression and disbelief when confronted by this enemy. That's why *Cancer Made Me Beautiful* is both timely and invaluable.

CHAPTER TWO

Exposing the Enemy

*"In all this you greatly rejoice, though now
for a little while you may have had to
suffer grief in all kinds of trials."*
1 Peter 1:6 (NIV)

The Journey Begins

2005 began differently than most years for me. That winter in Chicago was milder than usual, but cold nonetheless. I was in the process of familiarizing myself with a new community, as having recently moved to an area further south of the family home which had been located in Harvey, IL. It was a bitter-sweet move. Having to relinquish the home occupied by my family for over 40 years, I realized that the time had come. All of my other family members had now moved on, and the home was found to be too large and costly to maintain. The day before the move, the family gathered together in the home for what we called a final packing party. We reminisced over memories that took place in the home, but were never forgotten. We each had a different favorite memory that we spoke about as we walked through the entire house, entering areas that had not been looked upon for some of us in a long time. We remembered the good as well as bad times including some childhood disciplinary moments that ultimately made us who we are or aren't today. Truth be told, I would have to admit that most of the disciplinary moments centered on me, as I proved to be very curious during my childhood.

Packing of the home not only caused us to discover things that we had not seen in years, but made us remember things, that for some of us, had not been thought of in a very long time. We laughed, held back tears at times, and believe it or not; somehow became closer to one another. We ate pizza and chicken throughout the night, staying awake waiting on the movers to arrive the next morning to remove all of the cherished items we had collected over the years. Before locking the doors one last time, we toasted the home that embodied all of our past and celebrated each of our futures, believing that the best was yet to come.

Work at that time also proved to be unusual. I was employed by TASC (Treatment Alternatives for Safe Communities), a not-for-profit organization that provides behavioral health recovery management services for individuals with substance abuse and mental health disorders involved in or effected by systems such as criminal justice, courts or child welfare. I was facing challenges professionally for the first time that daily questioned my commitment and stamina. I found myself faced with the start-up of new programs inside of four separate correctional institutions throughout Chicago and its surrounding areas, one of which was under the watchful eye of the Governor's office. This was in addition to overseeing three other programs for individuals in Recovery as well as people impacted by HIV. You see, at the time, I was the Administrator of a unit housing all of these programs, responsible for staff and program accountability.

This was also the last year of high school for my nephew Jeremy, who is very important to me. My juggling act consisted of supporting him in his extra curricula school activities as well as managing program development and conflict at work. I found myself in my car for at least six hours a day, Monday thru Friday, just traveling from location to location. I remember my brother one day asking me, after seeming to always speak to me when I was in my car, what exactly did I do at my job? I responded "I'm a driver". We laughed and I kept driving.

Weekends did not lend themselves to a lot of relaxation either, since it involved spending time with one of the most important men in my life, my father. At the start of my journey in 2005 Dad was 86 years old. Spending time with him was at the top of my list of priorities and remained so throughout the writing process of this book. I believed it was very important that time be devoted to him since he no longer drove but still loved to get out. After my mother passed away in 1972 he became and remained the single parent who much of the credit for my family's success must be attributed. So to dedicate time out of my week to allow him to fulfill a little bit of his desires in life was the least I could do. Along with the fact that I have a lot of fun with my father, while still looking to him for wisdom.

I found myself on Sundays sitting in the pews of Trinity United Church of Christ, the church where I am a member, asking God, was all of this busyness necessary and what was it for? I received no response. But one morning, something unusual occurred that woke me from my sleep earlier than I had planned to arise. My clock radio went off playing a song entitled "He's Preparing Me", by Darryl Coley. I didn't think much of it at the time other than wondering why my clock was even going off at all. So I hit the snooze button and went back to sleep.

To most people alarm clocks are nothing unusual, but being retired Air Force and having experienced Basic Training, where being awakened abruptly every morning by reveille; left me never wanting to be awakened by any abrupt noise at all. Needless to say, I never used alarm clocks again. I learned that psychologically I could set my internal clock and it would awaken me naturally. So to hear my clock radio go off, not only irritated me, but also made me wonder when or who had set it. It actually crossed my mind that maybe Lonnetta had been messing with my radio, since we had begun to live together six months before.

In an attempt to get to the bottom of what was truly going on in my life and in some way reconcile my emotions and feelings with my day to day life, I signed up for bible courses at my church. Little did I know these classes would unlock a desire that I never realized had been hidden away in the recesses of my being, which was to understand the Bible for all of its possible meanings. The study of theology became my quest and I knew that Trinity UCC was exactly where I needed to be with Rev.

Dr. Jeremiah A. Wright, Jr. being an extraordinary theologian and teacher.

I had joined the family of Trinity 4 years prior, and for the first time in my church life found myself sitting in the pews taking notes during each of his sermons. Here was this man, this father, this husband, this minister, this pastor teaching and unfolding scripture in such a captivating manner that made me want to study to know more. For the first time I was hearing the scripture from a historical perspective that, as never before, allowed me to see my culture, my faith and amazingly, myself in the words. I began to forget about my day to day issues and thirsted for more and more information in the area of theology. But I will discuss this in more detail later.

It was now April and beginning to warm up outside. Winter coats were replaced by trench coats, and my commute between programs was becoming a bit more pleasant. One Wednesday evening after returning home from work, I played the messages on the answering service as I did most evenings, only to find a message from my doctor's office reminding me to schedule an appointment for my colonoscopy. Since my mother had passed away from colon cancer, I always knew, as did my doctor, the importance of this test every three years. So some time during the next day I called and scheduled the procedure and also made arrangements to be off work for the day of April 24, 2005.

Everyone 50 or older should be screened for colorectal cancer, or if you have a family history of the disease.

Colonoscopy is one method that your doctor can use to screen for colorectal cancer.

Cancer of the colon or rectum is also called colorectal cancer. In the United States, it is the fourth most common cancer in men and women. Caught early, it is often curable. It is more common in people over 50, and the risk increases with age. Since I was only 47 at the time I wasn't real concerned, although, this was the exact age of my mother's death from the disease. Still, I knew that you are more likely to get it if you have: 1) Polyps - growths inside the colon and rectum that may become cancerous, 2) A diet high in fat and 3) A family history or personal history of colorectal cancer   I wasn't sure about number one, but numbers two and three were definitely risk factors for me.

On April 24th I checked into the hospital as required after drinking the pre-op cleansing medicine which I took the previous day. No matter what they tell you about the taste, don't believe it. It is the hardest liquid to drink. The one tip that I can offer for this pre-opt process, is to have ginger ale on hand to help stomach it all.

After the procedure I was told that 2 polyps were removed and given a clean bill of health. So I left the hospital, as this was an outpatient procedure, with a full blown craving for a steak to replenish my red blood cells. But what happened in the upcoming months challenged me in ways that I could not have imagined.

Surviving the Trauma

It is now May 1, 2005. Work and my personal life seemed to ratchet up the stress level in ways that I had never experienced. Jeremy was in the last month of high-school with more and more activities requiring attendance. All of the correctional programs under my supervision were requiring more and more of my attention, while the program that I spoke of that was overseen by the Governor's office, seemingly began to fall apart. At one point, my superiors along with myself were called into the facility for a meeting. For the first time, my professional competence was brought into question.

The warden of the institution was asking for someone's head and for the first time in my career, I actually didn't care if it was mine. Ultimately the program was taken out of my department and given to another Administrator. I found myself standing outside of this ugly concrete structure that we call prison. And it occurred to me that this must be what it feels like for those inmates who had been wrongly accused. I asked God, "What was all of this really about?" Again I received no answer. Yet when I got into my car to drive home and turned to the radio station that I so regularly listened to, there was that song again "He's Preparing Me".

Around this time I was beginning to experience a numbing abdominal pain that was becoming constant. At first I assumed that the level of stress in my life was beginning to take a toll, which was so unlike me. But I thought, what else could it be? Still the pain continued. I returned to the doctor who had performed my colonoscopy to find out if something had gone wrong during the procedure.

After a quick examination, I was informed that I had a severe case of gas and prescribed medication. It was easy for me to accept this prognosis since with everything going on in my life proper nutrition had not been high on my list. Most of my meals were being consumed in my car or while sitting over a computer at night just to keep up.

By mid-May my gut and abdomen told me that the discomfort I was experiencing was not gas and required further diagnosis and investigation. So I made an appointment with my primary doctor for a more in-depth examination. At that time I had HMO insurance and became uniquely aware of why the fight for adequate health care through reform needed to be an undertaking in this country.

My primary doctor concurred with the surgical doctor and totally dismissed my concerns. She advised me to give the medication a chance to work, even though I had now been on the medication for over 2 weeks, (along with Advil as a secondary medication for the pain) with no relief. I was being made to feel as though my symptoms were psychological, for surely the doctors knew what they were talking about, or at least I thought they should. Nevertheless, the pain was not letting up.

I was now into the third week of pain, taking prescribed and over the counter medication and still attempting to keep up with everything in my day to day life. The pain had intensified to a level that forced me to leave work each day by 3pm in an effort to be in bed by 4pm. Nights found me preparing a tub of completely hot water to sit in, attempting to relieve the pain. The water could never get hot enough. It was then that I knew without a doubt, I had to take the lead in my own health care and press the doctors for more tests. This in itself became a very daunting experience that required all of my knowledge and skills of persuasion. Since with HMO insurance, a referral is required to see any other doctors, my primary physician found me to be a very formidable opponent in convincing her to schedule further testing for an accurate diagnosis. After much prodding and pressure from me, and maybe even a threat or two, a Cat-Scan was scheduled. This is where the trauma really began.

Again I entered the hospital through the out-patient facility, subjected this time to ingesting a liquid called barium that would allow for the doctors to have a better visual of what was really going on inside of me. Only this time I was not privileged, nor did I have access to ginger ale to help with the digestion of the fluid. Surprisingly, this day I felt the best that I had in a very long time. I began to think that maybe the light at the end of the tunnel was beginning to peak through. So I left the procedure to attend my nephew's performance in his school's Show Choir. The show ended around 8pm and the family went to dinner to congratulate Jeremy on a superior performance.

Upon returning home at approximately 10pm, from what I thought to be a good day; I received some very unexpected and unprepared for news. As someone once said, "It is always darkest before the dawn". Well after listening to my answering service, the sun truly went down for me. Actually it felt more like an eclipse.

While retrieving messages, five of them were from the technician who performed my CAT-scan urgently requesting that I return to the hospital. He stated that my appendix was at least 3 times the normal size and that an eruption was imminent. He also informed me that my physician was waiting on a call from me to further explain my condition and he proceeded to give me her home number. For the first time, I knew what it felt like to be sucker-punched.

Calling my primary physician proved to be very disappointing, yet eye opening; providing a glimpse into the challenges when working with the medical profession. While my doctor agreed with the technician's message and the nature of his call, she was angry that he'd called alerting me to a potential emergency. I was confused and then appalled when she shared that the basis of her anger was because she was going on a long weekend trip with her family and wanted my admission to wait until the next week. This was one of the most difficult things for me to hear, as it was in total conflict with what I believed or understood about physicians' code of conduct. Again, control of my own health care had to be in my hands.

Against my primary physician's desires, I followed the advice of the technician and checked into the hospital that night. I'm sure that my primary physician, afraid of the potential outcome, decided to make the referral and meet me at the hospital, but performed no examination of any kind. I had no doubt that this assertive move on my part motivated her to make the referral and at least meet me at the hospital. I explained to her that this was not my preference for a weekend outing for myself either.

It was at that moment I made the decision to terminate my relationship with my primary doctor as soon as possible.

I was admitted into the hospital flanked by my sisters and friends concerned for my health. We all fully expected that I would be wheeled into emergency surgery before day-break. But to our surprise, the only precaution taken that night, for what was reportedly an imminent appendix rupture, was an I.V started with morphine. Throughout the night there were no examinations or discussions with a physician; only my primary physician, who merely signed the admissions papers. We were left to wonder what type of emergency could this have really been or was my delay in care based on other factors.

It wasn't until the next morning that I finally saw a doctor who attempted to shed some light on my health challenges. He was the surgeon who had been called in because of an alleged diagnosis of an appendix rupture. He proceeded to inform me that he was not removing my appendix, as it had not been affected, nor was it the cause of my pain. Imagine my dismay. Unaccustomed to the drug morphine, I first thought that I was not hearing him correctly, so I looked to my sisters for clarity. When they confirmed that what I thought I heard, was actually what I did hear, I then felt as if I was having a bad nightmare that was just beginning.

The next physician to come into my room was my primary. She introduced me to a gastrologist. I'm convinced that she did this because she couldn't and wouldn't admit that her original diagnosis of gas was wrong. The gastrologist proceeded to order more medical tests, sure that he could get to the bottom of what was really going on. That evening however, I looked up in surprise, only to see my gynecologist enter my room.

One might ask, why my gynecologist? But because I trusted her and had a good relationship with her, I was glad to see someone that would tell me the truth. Even if the simple truth at that point was only to say that they did not know what was wrong with me.

She apparently saw the fear and confusion on my face and immediately wheeled me out of what I referred to then as the pit of hell. She took me to a private examination room on the same floor first talking to me woman to medical woman about what was going on. She then examined me fully and informed me that fibroids had been identified. Yet, in her opinion fibroids were not likely the real source of my extreme pain. We talked for a while longer and together decided to perform a partial hysterectomy in the next couple of days hoping, but not convinced that this would be the cure I so desperately sought. She had only one concern about performing such a procedure; my lack of ever giving birth. I assured her that at my age, this was not a concern and that I had given up on the dream of being a biological mother and had since placed the idea into the unanswered dream column of my life. I was however, very appreciative that she considered my feelings before making such an important decision, particularly since up to this point every other medical professional seemed to discount my assessment or feelings, even though I was the person experiencing the discomfort.

The next day involved one test after another that had been recommended by the gastrologist. I was poked and prodded in areas I didn't even know existed. I was awakened for my temperature and other vitals. I was awakened to decide what meals I wanted. But the most appalling for me was being awakened to be given something to help me sleep. It all left me anxious to leave the hospital. I even found myself looking forward to my sister Lonnetta's cooking. That in itself spoke volumes about how much I wanted out of the hospital.

As I awoke the next morning the gastrologist entering my room to give me the prognosis from the previous day's battery of tests. What he told me shook me to my core. He informed me that I had Crohn's Disease and that medication would be needed for the remainder of my life. I felt as though he had given me a life sentence diagnosis. And on some level, I'm sure I shut down and started imagining the worst.

Once I pulled myself together and started to come back to reality, I phoned my sister and asked her to go on-line, research Crohn's disease and bring me everything she could find. The first thing that I read was that Crohn's disease is an inflammatory bowel disease (IBD). It causes inflammation of the lining of your digestive tract, which can lead to abdominal pain, severe diarrhea and even malnutrition.

The inflammation caused by Crohn's disease often spreads deep into the layers of affected bowel tissue. Like ulcerative colitis, another common IBD, Crohn's disease can be both painful and debilitating and sometimes may lead to life-threatening complications.

While there's no known medical cure for Crohn's disease, therapies can greatly reduce the signs and symptoms of the disease and even bring about long-term remission. With these therapies, many people with Crohn's disease are able to function well.

Although these symptoms seemed to explain what was going on with me, my spirit denied the diagnosis, but I was unsure what to do next. So I began the medication and prepared for my next procedure (partial hysterectomy) to take place in five days.

In the meantime, I returned to work for the next few days to prepare staff for my absence and wrap up any professional loose ends, all while trying to wrap my head around and accept the diagnosis that I had been given. I scheduled appointments with all the programs under my supervision to inform them that I would be away for a minimum of six weeks, however, I would begin working from home the last three weeks of my leave. But as someone once said, "You plan and God laughs".

The time had come for my hysterectomy. There I was checking into the hospital, but this time not as an outpatient. Again I sat in the lobby waiting to be called to show my insurance card to the hospital clerk. Again I was giving my birthdate, social security number and address as if it had all changed in one week. I sat with my overnight bag in tow with only my toiletries, slippers and a change of clothes to return home in. I was now experienced enough to know that sleepwear was not needed nor could it be used in hospitals. But only as I can, my pillow and comforter were also with me. Not to mention that I'm convinced that it's the hospitals goal to make you as uncomfortable as possible. They provide paper thin blankets while freezing you to death by blowing sub-zero air conditioning the entire time. I was having none of that.

> *"When you pass through the waters, I will be with you, and through the rivers, they shall not overwhelm you, when you walk through the fire, you shall not be burned, nor shall the flame scorch you"*
>
> **ISAIAH 43:2 (NKJV)**

My sisters and best friend were with me, but had no idea of the concerns that were swirling around in my head. As usual I put on a brave front as only I could. I knew that I had said my prayers morning, noon and night prior to this moment and somewhere deep in the recesses of my soul, I felt that this was one of those trials or tests Pastor Wright spoke of so often from the pulpit. But for some reason, now that the reality of surgery was here, coming from a long line of prayer warriors didn't help. All I could think to say was "Precious Lord take my hand".

The other statement that came to mind was "Thy will be done," a statement I found to be easier said than believed, especially when you have no idea what his will is for you. It is also difficult when you don't feel that you have been the best child of God that you could or should have been throughout your life; not to mention the past few years.

But you say it and silently pray (or are we really trying to bargain at that time) that his will is something that you can handle.

While waiting to be called for service, I opened my bible and took comfort in Isaiah 43:2 that says *"When you pass through the waters, I will be with you, and through the rivers, they shall not overwhelm you, when you walk through the fire, you shall not be burned, nor shall the flame scorch you"* (NKJV). Although I had never deconstructed this verse in relationship to my own life, my spirit told me to marinate over these words for the peace I so desperately sought.

It was time for the surgery. I was wheeled off to pre-op, given the drugs for relaxation, shaved and prepared for surgery. Once wheeled off into the surgical area, I had to leave behind all of the faces (family and friends) I loved. This is one of those life situations that you do alone, no sharing, no familiar voice of loved ones saying everything will be alright, no familiar touch of support to give you courage. This is the time that your relationship with God intensifies and if you listen real closely with your spiritual ear, his voice becomes audible and comforting. It is then you learn the meaning of resting in his arms.

> *"...love, not work; love, not money; love, not possessions, is the most important thing in life."*

Surgery was now complete and I regained consciousness in the recovery room. Opening my eyes and being coherent enough to know what I was seeing, I woke to the faces of my family and friends. This indicated to me that I had made it through the surgery safely. The healing could finally begin. But wait, I remembered that I was still diagnosed with Crohn's disease for which there was no cure. So for a while, my much anticipated joy was replaced by depression. I was discharged within 24 hours with the regular post-op instructions for recovery. But little did I know, a ray of light had broken through, even though I couldn't see it. For it was and still is my belief that this seemingly unnecessary hysterectomy revealed what was really there inside of me, calling out to be identified, to surface in a way that would or could no longer be ignored.

I was taken home where my comfort and health took top prority for my family, with my Lonnetta being my primary caregiver. To avoid going up and down the stairs to my 2nd floor bedroom, a day bed was placed in the dining room allowing me to rest during the day. Lonnetta in turn, was convinced that I had to eat healthy, even though most of what she came up with made me nauseous. Our taste buds are not really compatible and neither is she the best of cooks. Yet I loved her for all that she did.

During her work hours there was a constant parade of family and friends poised to check on me and cater to my every whim, whether I felt like company or not. But these are the times that you come to realize that love, not work; love, not money; love, not possessions, are the most important things in life. So whatever depression attempted to seep in was replaced by thanksgiving and gratitude.

I had now been home for two days, but comfort eluded me as each day passed. Someone told me that walking would help when recovering from a hysterectomy. So by day three, around 4am, I began to walk in circles through the living room, dining room and kitchen. I said goodbye to Lonnetta as she headed off to work trying to appear as if all was well as not to worry her, but feeling that something was gravely wrong.

At approximately 9am my Godson Kenyatta, who had moved to the area six months prior in response to an employment opportunity, arrived right around the time that nausea took hold of me in a major way. I believed that the feeling I was experiencing had nothing to do with the surgery just performed. I phoned the gastrologist who had diagnosed Crohn's and explained my symptoms to him, which apparently alarmed him as well. He instructed me to meet him at the hospital immediately for examination. So there I was again, headed to the hospital. I felt as though the doctors were cruelly making up for all of the 47 years of my life when I had been healthy and never spent a day in the hospital.

Seeing the fear and worry in my godson's eyes, I instructed him to call my friend Dorothy who lived nearby, to accompany us. I knew as a young man in his twenties, he was likely terrified by the potential medical emergency and decisions that might emerge. Plus, if he was anything like my father and brother, the thought of female issues made him uncomfortable.

Dorothy and Kenyatta took me to the hospital while phoning my family on the way. I could see the fear in their eyes as none of us knew what was really wrong or what to expect. This particular trip to the hospital proved to be the worst yet. For the first time I felt gravely ill, in pain and unable to fight for myself. But I trusted that after my sister Lonnetta arrived, my rights and needs would be given the priority deserved. For what people didn't know about my family was that over the years, caring for my father through strokes, a pulmonary embolism, a heart attack, two shunts due to cerebral hematoma and other medical emergencies; we had become quite adept at navigating hospitals and the medical profession at large.

I was admitted into the hospital, but this time with doctors afraid of not getting it right. Finally, hopefully, prayerfully; the real cause of my pain would be identified. I was placed on a morphine drip again, along with vicodin 3 times daily. And because the pain had now become unbearable, if the two medications were administered close to each other, there were times that I felt myself go into another orbit. Nevertheless, I was determined to stay alert in an effort to manage my health care effectively. For obvious reasons, I didn't trust the medical professionals to do what was right. I made my own decision to immediately discontinue the Crohn's medication, hiding the pills in the bedside drawer. For as I stated earlier, I never believed it to be an accurate diagnosis, which finally proved to be the case.

On Day 3 of my stay the doctor walked in only to confirm my beliefs. Crohn's disease was not the enemy I was at war with. The doctor proceeded to tell me that all indications were pointing to something he referred to as Lymphoma. He was bringing in an oncologist to perform a biopsy and a bone marrow test to confirm his suspicions. As I stated in the introduction, I knew nothing about Lymphoma, nor, that it was a form of cancer. So again I asked my sister for information on lymphoma, just as I had requested on Crohn's disease. I intended to study and develop any pertinent questions for the oncologist before he arrived.

That night found me to be very restless while at times questioning my faith. I had moved from one disease to another in a matter of hours. I wasn't even sure of what prayer to say or what exactly to pray for. My mind reeled between what to think, and what to expect. A numbness of sorts engulfed me making the night seem much longer than it was. By day-break, I was exhausted from my own thoughts and could only think to call out to God for understanding. I will be the first to admit that when the odds seem overwhelming; our situations can threaten to obscure God's personal revelation for us. It is in these moments that our circumstances seem hopeless and our "normal" way of living, praying and believing don't seem to be effective. But it is also in these moments that we must permit our faith to reach past our wounds and hurts and take hold of the healing and delivering power of the infinite realm of possibility in Jesus Christ. So again I rested in his arms.

As scheduled, the oncologist arrived the next morning and I was wheeled off to the surgical area yet again to have a biopsy performed. This is a procedure that involves the removal of cells or tissues so they can be viewed under a microscope to check for signs of cancer. The doctor may remove a growth from the skin, if there is one; to be examined by a pathologist. But my growth was internal which caused for a different type of procedure.

Looking back, this had to have been the most painful procedure throughout my entire journey, although necessary to arrive at a correct diagnosis. Not to mention, that while a painful test, anesthesia cannot be administered since the patient has to be awake and able to respond to the physician.

I was made to lay on my stomach, directly where the source of all of my pain emanated from, while the doctor entered through by back, past my spine, down through to my abdomen to extract a piece of tissue from the affected area. I'm not sure how long the procedure took, although they assured me that it was a short period of time. To me, it felt like I had aged an entire year without celebrating any holidays and that I was being punished for everything that I had done wrong in my life.

Even though the nurse attempted to comfort me through the ordeal, I felt like slapping her every time she leaned in to assure me that I was doing great. All I could think of was that she knew nothing of the pain I was experiencing, thus I needed her to be silent. It's like when someone says to you, I know exactly how you feel, when in reality they haven't a clue.

The next day the oncologist arrived with the results of the biopsy. It was official. I had Lymphoma Cancer. The real diagnosis for my pain was finally reached. The enemy had been exposed.

CHAPTER THREE

The Dance

*"I know what it is to be in need, and I know what
it is to have plenty. I have learned the secret of
being content in any and every situation, whether
well fed or hungry, whether living in plenty or in
want. I can do everything through him who
gives me strength".*
Philippians 4:12-13 (NIV)

To dance -- to live in a way that is consistent with our longing. To dance, alone or with others, is to live authentically as we attempt to live out our purpose. To do this, we must learn how to reconcile or let go of the past and slow down and embrace the present, returning to our First Love (God) where we encounter our true self.

Reconciling the Past

When the doctor walked in with the diagnosis of Lymphoma, I thought that I was prepared to hear everything that he had to say. I had compiled a list of questions from all I had read as well as treatment possibilities I had discussed with my sisters. And yet, all I heard out of his mouth was cancer. I closed my eyes and thought "the thing that I feared the most had now come upon me", which was to be diagnosed with cancer just like my mother. But I never thought that when my diagnosis came, I would be exactly the same age she was when she lost her battle with this enemy.

At that moment I was transported back to when I was 15 years old. It was if I was reliving being told that my mother would not recover from colon cancer.

The year was 1972 and my family lived in Harvey, IL. I was 15, my sisters Denise and Lonnetta were 17 and 18 respectively and then there was Lonnie my brother, he was 7 years of age. Lonnetta was preparing to go off to college for her second year, while Denise floated throughout the house ready to embark upon her first. My excitement existed because one of my favorite holidays, Labor Day, was about to be celebrated.

I loved summer holidays since this was the time that dad grilled ribs, chicken, potatoes and corn in the backyard and homemade ice cream was made instead of store bought. There is nothing like homemade ice cream from one of the old time ice cream machines that you had to manually crank and add whatever flavor you liked. But the flavor of choice for my family was always vanilla. This particular holiday also included parades and outside games. Since I was a tomboy softball was my game of choice, but I also enjoyed basketball and jump rope as well, now having the knees to prove it.

During summer holidays and cookouts, my parents always partnered with the next door neighbor who had children the same age as each of my sisters and brother. You see, this was an era when families were part of a community. The rearing of children was accomplished by all of the community's adults. I wanted to say elders, but since I am now the age my parents were then, I not only view the word elder differently, I would like to think that I am not in that age group. To use the word elders referring to my parents at that time would mean that I am an elder now. I'm not sure that I am ready for that title at this juncture in my life, except when I want my brother, nephew and god-children to do as I say. What I also did not realize then, but do now, is that families, because of their commitment to the upbringing and success of the overall community, joined together at these times as not to have to shoulder the entire expense for occasions such as cookouts allowing for families to enjoy what the season had to offer.

But at age 15, mostly this was a time that we were given permission to drink pop (soda), eat cake and sweets without having our eating habits monitored. You see soda was reserved for guests in our home no matter the flavor, and only my mom was able to drink the little bottles of Coca Cola, and she did by the case. We later learned that cocaine was an ingredient in those small bottles. Children during that time, were made to drink milk, Kool-Aid, juice or water. So in one aspect, holidays meant freedom to me. More than that, this was the last holiday before returning to school.

This particular Labor Day mom wasn't feeling very well,

but as she always did, she pushed through it. She had returned from a vacation with our cousin to Spain and Africa the month before. The trip was the result of a year's worth of saving. She had us all convinced that she was suffering from having eaten something that didn't agree with her while out of the country. So of course, we didn't give it much thought and went on with the day as normal.

The day following the Labor Day of 1972 changed my family's life forever. While we knew that mom wasn't feeling well, we were not in any way prepared for what came next.

Mom woke with her stomach bloated as if she were 8 months pregnant. Dad informed us that they needed to go to the hospital. When he returned home my mother was not with him and we were told that she was more ill than we thought and surgery would have to be performed. Still the idea of losing my mother had not entered my mind. At the age of 15 you expect to have your mother with you forever, or at least until you're grown. Plus, at that time I didn't know anyone who had lost their mother to death or maybe I had been shielded from that information prior to that point in life. But the shield was soon to be shattered.

My mother was everything to my family. She was the mother, disciplinarian, cook, housekeeper, seamstress, counselor and comforter. My father relied on her for everything, as did we, for all pertaining to the upkeep and running of the home, including listening to our problems and encouraging us when we thought we came up short. She was the first one who ever told me that I could do or be anything I wanted. She always had a way of imparting words of wisdom without you feeling lectured to.

The community saw her as the Sunday School teacher, bible scholar, PTA leader, gospel singer and mother to all. Our friends felt that they could talk to my mother as well, even when their own parents didn't listen. I literally thought that my mother knew everything. So in my head, I rationalized that there was no way that the God that I thought I knew, would take such a woman from us all and especially me.

My mother remained in the hospital for months and we were told that she had colon cancer. Still the thought of losing her was not my reality. To deal with her illness seemed to be just a difficult phase for the family.

Mom came home once during her illness. During that time we turned one of the bedrooms into a hospital room, bed and all. These changes never fazed me, nor did I think that these would be the last months that she would spend in our home. All I knew was that I had my mother back to talk to everyday.

Then the unthinkable happened. Her illness became worse and her return to the hospital inevitable. The last time that my mom returned to the hospital, culminated in her eventually slipping into a coma. The mother that I knew and loved was no more. She was 47 years old when she lost her battle with colon cancer, at 3am on July 20, 1972, which was also my brother's 8th birthday.

Knowing that my father had also lost his mother at age

seven, I had always prayed that history would not repeat itself. Even though mom had been ill during my brother's entire 7th year, I thought that we would have more time before the angel of death issued such an impacting blow to the family. I found myself unable to reconcile my faith with what was going on in my reality.

After being told by church leaders all of my life that God heals and answers prayers, I naturally wondered why my prayers weren't answered and my mother healed. At the age of 16, one tends to take the scripture literally and believe exactly what is being said. No one explained that God's will does not always match up to our will and could sometimes be totally contradictory to what we want or expect. Needless to say, I wasn't very happy with God during that period of my life. And because my mother had made it her life's work to convince us to read for knowledge, as I aged, I began to view all of the books that promoted positive thinking and seeing the glass half full; as crap. Sermons conducted by ministers that taught prayer for healing, began to grate on my nerves. What were they saying? Had we prayed wrong? Did we not use the right words? Was my mother not worthy of healing? None of it made sense to me any longer.

All that I could focus on during that season was that I felt left behind by my sisters, (Lonnetta returning to college and Denise heading to Germany to join her new husband) alone at home to care for an 8 year old and a father who worked nights. I was expected to complete high school, oversee my brother's schooling and run a household; all without the guidance of my mother. I knew that if I was to do this, high school had to be completed quickly. So

I enrolled in night classes to obtain additional credits, graduating in 3 years instead of 4; moving on to college, all before my 17th birthday.

For a while I began to think that I could live life on my own terms. My life became consumed with chaos and regret, but mostly I lived a life consumed with grief; no one ever seeing the pain inside. Not knowing that I was carrying a level of anger that would eventually have to be dealt with I continued, what I considered, the ritual act of attending church on a regular basis, wearing the mask and perfecting the act of a woman of faith. Along the way, somehow I began to learn the lesson that "bad things happen to good people"; while yet to understand or accept that God is sovereign and can do what he wants, when he wants, and how he wants; all the while having the best for me in mind. Eventually I came to embrace this truth.

I reopened my eyes at this point, only to remember that I was the one laying in the hospital bed being told that this time it was me being invaded by cancer. I began to cry for the first time realizing that I was exactly the same age (47) as my mother when she died of cancer. I again asked God why. And yet again, no answer. But just as the tears began to fall, I remembered a scripture that my mother quoted regularly and even had a plaque engraved for each of us that read, *"Trust in the Lord with all your heart, and lean not on your own understanding. In all your ways acknowledge him, and he will direct your path"* Proverbs 3:5 NIV. I then heard my mother's voice for the first time since her death, telling me "God did not give you a spirit of fear" and that my healing would come, in a tone that could only be my mom, Augusta Hunter.

On one level I received what she said with joy. On the other hand, strangely enough anger also accompanied it. Since her death I had asked to see or hear from her in a dream or any other manner, and it had not happened. Now here she was speaking to me, just as I wanted, and I was questioning where she had been all these years. Nevertheless I was able to reconcile my anger with the joy I felt knowing that there was no better time than this for her to speak to me, and I found myself smiling despite my circumstances. Right then I remembered the scripture that I had read just before my surgery earlier that month that says *"When you pass through the waters, I will be with you, and through the rivers, they shall not overwhelm you, when you walk through the fire, you shall not be burned, nor shall the flame scorch you."* Isaiah 43:2 (NKJV). For the first time, I felt that just maybe, she along with God, had been watching over me all these years, not feeling the need to speak to me until now.

I must confess that even this did not totally prevent fear from setting in on some level. Even though it was 2005, I grew up in an era that Cancer was referred to as the Big C, and ultimately death. Remember, it took my mother from my family and me. So emotionally and mentally, I felt that I was coming face to face with my own mortality.

It was then that I rejoined the conversation with the oncologist and heard him say that a final test (a bone marrow) must be performed to determine the type and stage of lymphoma I had and whether or not the cancer had entered my bones.

A bone marrow test is when a physician conducts a procedure to collect and examine bone marrow — the spongy tissue inside some of our larger bones. A bone marrow biopsy reveals whether the bone marrow is healthy and making normal amounts of blood cells. Doctors use bone marrow biopsy to diagnose and monitor blood and marrow diseases, including some cancers.

I found my voice just enough to ask the questions that were stuck in my throat, wrapped in fear. What would it mean if my bones had been affected, and what were my chances for recovery? I can't tell you that I heard a lot of what he said at that moment, except for the fact that my recovery rate could stand at 95% if the bone had not been penetrated. I trusted that my sisters caught everything else that had been spoken by the doctor. Again, all I could do was lay back and rest in the arms of Jesus.

So the test was scheduled for the next morning. And eventually, everyone left me alone to confront my own doubts and fears throughout the night.

Now that I had digested at least on some level, my prognosis, my mind turned to my father. How could I tell him that I had cancer? How could I tell him that while I was busy the last few years taking care of him, the enemy that he loathed had returned to attack his youngest daughter? How could I allow him to feel the possibility of another loss to this disease that he had come to hate and ultimately blame for the loss of his wife? Even though I wanted nothing more than for him to hug me and call me 'Honeybunch' as he did when I was a child and tell me everything would be ok, how could I be the cause of him at age 86, having to confront what was now seen as our family's most formidable opponent.

So it was then that my sisters and I made a pact. Dad was not to know the real reason of my illness. My brother was now living in New Jersey, so a phone call was placed to him as well, to ensure that it didn't come up in conversation during their regular father-son phone conversations. I actually didn't divulge the word cancer to my father until treatment was completed and I knew that the cancer was defeated. I knew that being a man, and especially at his age, if I said female problems, he wouldn't ask any more questions; because this was a subject he didn't like to discuss. And since he was accustomed to me changing my hair style on a regular basis, I knew that he wouldn't give a second thought to seeing me in a wig. To be honest, the writing of this book, and being able to read it to him before his death (February 8, 2011) was the first glimpse for him into what that period of time really held for me regarding my health challenges. Surprisingly, he turned out to be my biggest supporter, pushing me to complete this book, by telling me that the world deserved to know my story.

Living in the Now
The following morning as I prepared for the doctor to arrive for my next procedure, I completed my morning meditation. I must admit that this was one of the most difficult and emotional prayer times ever.

I then spoke with the nurse on duty since by now we had become friendly and she seemed to sympathize with my plight. Having just gone through what I considered to be torture the day before with the biopsy, I asked her to be prepared to administer my morphine shot as soon as the doctor arrived on the floor and that I would also take my vicodin at the same time. I figured that if I had to be awake during the procedure, I would numb myself enough to make me void of any feeling.

What I was not prepared for was that the procedure would be done in my room. And even though the doctor explained that the procedure would be quick and simple, both my sister Denise (my support for this time of the day), and I were caught off guard when she was encouraged to remain in the room.

While standing by my bedside and holding my hand, Denise was able to observe upclose; when the physician cut my hip bone and removed the small piece of bone needed for assessment. Since I had not made her privy to my plan of "numbing" myself prior to the procedure, she became very concerned about my seemingly lack of feeling. She began to demand that I say something about how I was feeling and I realized even through my dazed state, that she would be the one that would have to be comforted through the process. For the first time throughout this entire ordeal, I was able to think of someone else, comfort someone else and care for someone else; instead of me. And I found myself more than happy to rise to the occasion.

All necessary tests had now been completed and the findings indicated that I had Non-Hodgkin's Lymphoma. Finally, I knew what was wrong, where the pain was coming from and that a cure was possible. I can't explain it, but at that moment Cancer didn't sound so bad on the heels of being told that I had Crohn's, an incurable and debilitating disease. I actually found myself feeling relieved, since this new diagnosis opened up the possibility of getting better. All that was left to do, was to decide the best treatment plan to accomplish the healing.

Remember the song I kept hearing at the beginning of my journey, "He's Preparing Me"? Well the words came back to me at that moment in full verse. "He's Preparing Me for something that I cannot handle right now. He's making me ready, just because he cares; He's providing me with what I'll need to carry out the next battle in my life." I finally understood why this song kept standing out over all other songs when I listened to the radio.

What became clear to me at that moment was that if I had not gone through everything that I had to get to this moment of a cancer diagnosis, and if given the correct diagnosis initially, I could not have handled it. I now knew that every moment in my journey, up to this point was meant to strengthen me and prepare me for not only the diagnosis; but ultimately the battle with the disease we call Cancer. I knew that while I felt that God had gone silent on me, while I was crying out at every turn, his angels had been dispatched all around me for comfort and protection, to include my own mother. But as they say, the teacher never speaks during test time. And oh what a test I had taken. However, the final exam looked like it could be open book if I wanted it to.

I heard someone once say that if you see yourself as a victim, you would only complain and see what's wrong. But, if you see yourself as a survivor, you would find the courage to stand, fight and want to make a difference. So I set out to accept the space that I was in, or should I say my present reality. I immediately began to see myself as a survivor even before treatment started. I knew that the most important challenge would be my mindset. I figured that by seeing a positive ending

When you are in battle, you must be ever vigilant, standing guard, but more than anything you have to know your enemy.

at the beginning of the treatment process, true healing could happen.

The form of treatment decided on for my cure was chemotherapy (also called chemo) for two days every three weeks for six months. Chemo is a type of cancer treatment using drugs to destroy cancer cells. It works by stopping or slowing the growth of cancer cells in the body. Chemotherapy is used for one of three purposes; to cure cancer, control cancer or to ease cancer symptoms. I was going for the Cure.

I swallowed hard and scheduled my first treatment to begin 4 days after release from the hospital. I must admit, I thought that maybe I would be given more time between diagnosis and the start of treatment, but my oncologist wanted to get started with my cure immediately. He stated that he felt me to be too young and vibrant to linger in the world of cancer any longer than necessary. I saw this as promising, remembering that the voice of my mother had said "my healing would come". So I gathered my internal strength, put a little makeup on my face and prepared to return home.

Upon release from the hospital, I was given a prescription for more vicodin as well as morphine patches to be applied every three days. You see, even though the correct diagnosis had been reached, my level of pain was still what I would only categorize as extreme. But it is interesting the level of pain that you can endure once its source is identified. Don't get me wrong, I did need the medication for pain.

I woke the next morning, finally in my own bed, and arose to shower. For the first time in a while I focused on what I looked like in the mirror. I had lost weight, but most of all muscle. I actually looked sick and this took me aback, as any major illness had managed to elude me my entire life. For the first time during this journey, I actually looked like I felt and I didn't like what I saw. My body looked vulnerable and weak, totally contradictory to what and who my spirit was telling me I was. The weight loss however, separate from the muscle loss was no problem, since I came to the table needing to lose a few pounds anyway. But this is not the weight loss program that I would recommend to anyone.

The next few days, before going to the Cancer Care Center that my oncologist was associated with and where I would be receiving my chemotherapy, I decided to embark upon an in-depth research of the cancer attacking my body. I believed that knowledge was power, and I intended to possess as much power as I could over this thing called cancer. This time, unlike when my mother battled and lost to this physical enemy, I believed that research and technology had advanced in such a way that would allow my fight to be different. During this time I thought of the song "I am on the Battlefield" and concluded that when you are in battle, you must be ever vigilant, standing guard; but more than anything you have to know your enemy.

I went on-line and printed everything there. The results of my study are described in Chapter One, under Lymphoma as a Type. I visited the library to read books written by others who had been stricken with Lymphoma. I spoke with a nutritionist and licensed master fitness trainer, (which I am one myself). Finally, I developed a list of questions for the oncologist to ask during my first appointment. When I entered the Cancer Center for my first treatment, I was fully armed with information and questions I required answers to. Every blood test, I requested copies of, as well as asking the nurse to teach me how to read them. I knew that this was my fight and I intended on winning it.

Even though I didn't fully know what to expect from chemotherapy, understanding that every patient reacts differently; not knowing how it would make me feel or whether or not it would work, the one thing I knew was that I really didn't want a port inserted into my chest that would remain for a year. A port is a surgically placed central or pick line in your body to permit easy access for blood draws or medicine injection without using your veins. So I arrived for treatment armed with the correct terminology, research and self-confidence, determined to convince my oncologist to use the veins in my arms when administering what they call your cocktail (mixture of drugs) through an IV. To my surprise, after much conversation and what I saw as impressing him with my knowledge, he agreed to my plan. Now I had to pray that my veins held up, as on a good day my veins are difficult to locate even to draw blood. But lo and behold, my veins stood up like little soldiers, even though at the end of all treatments, I looked as if I had tracks in my arms. Then my prayer became that I would not be stopped by the police while driving, as they would think that I was an addict. The truth, unknown at the beginning however, was that I was becoming addicted to all of the pain medication. But I will talk about that in the next chapter.

> *This fight calls for a little more than just praying and crying. It calls for us to fight while praying and crying.*

The best thing about treatment to me, was receiving Benadryl through the IV first before any other drug. The purpose of the Benadryl was to ensure that I had no adverse reactions to subsequent drugs administered during treatment. But that was not why I liked it. To most, I'm sure that this sounds crazy, but to someone such as myself, who had never used this drug for allergies, I found it to be the best sleep aid ever. I began to look forward to my treatments just for the sleep experience. But as with any drug, the body adapts and the reaction changes. So by treatment number three (week nine), I remained awake and began to interact with the other patients.

Receiving treatment in a cancer care center as opposed to a doctor's office means you are not alone. You are joined by others receiving treatment from various forms and stages of cancer. Most often you are scheduled with the same group of individuals on an ongoing basis. This made me the newbie of the group my first couple of weeks of treatment, not to mention that I had a lower level of comfort when speaking about my illness. However, anyone who knows me, knows that it didn't take long before I became fully engaged in conversation.

Conversing with what I began to refer to as my colleagues in the field of cancer survival, became an unexpected blessing. There we all were; young, old, black, white, male and female. We came from all walks of life, income levels and professions, but we quickly realized that this was a disease that had no respect of person. We shared our thoughts, fears and experiences, and became our own unofficial support group. Through the interaction with my peers, and as I accepted the fact that no one was exempt; I began to shift from the question Why me, to Why not me? Plus, it wasn't as if my life had been pure or that I had not participated in drinking, smoking and other unhealthy habits during my earlier years. Remember, I said earlier that after my mom's death I did everything that I thought I was big and bad enough to do. Ultimately, our support group came to know that a fight was going on, and we had to get in it, no matter our past discretions.

Think about the song by Donnie McClurken "Stand". He

says, "when you have done all that you can do, then you stand". For me this song tells us that there is work to be done on our part as well. And this fight calls for a little more than just praying and crying. It calls for us to fight while praying and crying; to know and understand who we are and whose we are; to know our opponent and what it would take to defeat it; and finally to come out of our comfort zones, putting on our battle gear, realizing we are on the front line now, prepared to take a few hits, but determined to win.

One of the most troubling things for me about treatment was the inevitability of losing my hair. Not because of vanity, but because it meant that others would realize my illness and not treat me the same. I thought of all the times that I had conducted training on stigma relating to HIV and ex-offenders, and for the first time realized that stigma affects us all on one level or another. I now knew that we all fear being stigmatized for something most often, out of our control; which keeps us from removing our mask and living an authentic life.

I had never been one to wear wigs. But after the second treatment, as I sat on the side of my bed one morning seeing several of my braids on my pillow; I took a deep breath, picked up the scissors and razor and headed into the bathroom. I felt that if I was to lose my hair, I would be the one to take it. So there I was, standing in the mirror, being my own barber, without ever having taken one course; cutting and shaving my head, while uncontrollable tears ran down my face. I stood at the end, seeing this bald-headed woman, thinner than usual and not a muscle in sight, wondering what else this journey held for me.

I never said that taking control of my situation or standing in my own power wasn't painful however, I found myself still thanking God for his grace and mercies allowing me to still be here. Knowing that even though the reflection in the mirror wasn't what I wanted for myself, I was still standing. Plus a good cry is healthy every now and then, or so I've heard.

My nephew Jeremy had by now graduated from high school and was off to college. His univeristy offered a program that permitted him to register early allowing for an easier transition for new students. My sisters asked if I could travel with them over an extended weekend for the family orientation and I agreed, as did my doctor. My close friend Dorothy, who is also the mother of two of my godsons, Vincent and Andrew; had also agreed to accompany us on this excursion. This would be an eight hour road trip one way. All I could say was "God be with us".

My concern was not my illness as much as it was about putting all of the personalities of my family and friend into one vehicle for that length of time. Even though we travel a lot together, road trips don't always work out very well. With each of us believing that we are the best drivers, coupled with us all having our own control issues, eight hours could feel like a lifetime. Just a simple food stop could take a 30 minute conversation to make a decision. And even with that, we would still stop at more than one location to satisfy everyone. But this time I had a secret weapon. My morphine patches and vicodin pills would permit me to zone out, preventing any expectations of me to weigh in on any heated and often emotional discussions. To my surprise the trip was enjoyable and we were all still speaking when we returned home. I actually think that harmony prevailed out of their concern for my health, so I tried to think of what I could tell them prior to future trips that would encourage this behavior to repeat itself.

Overall, the trip proved that it was time for me to develop a plan for returning to work. Up until now, it was easy to face family and friends, but I had to prepare myself for what I saw as the public at large. Remember, I was Administrator of programs within a human services agency that focused on drug and alcohol recovery and re-entry for ex-offenders. So, having the look or demeanor of "woe is me" was not an option. I had to figure out a way to disguise my pain or any signs of exhaustion, since I knew that staff as well as the people we served, looked to me to offer a ray of hope. So needless to say, my prayer and meditation time increased; as did my walking time in an effort to increase my energy level.

After much planning and reflection, I spoke with my doctor, made a call to the HR department of the company and set a date to return to work.

CHAPTER FOUR

Wholeness:
Recovery on all Levels

*"So we do not lose heart; Even though our outer
nature is wasting away, our inner nature is being
renewed day by day. For this slight momentary
affliction is preparing us for an eternal weight of
glory beyond measure. For we look not at what can
be seen, but at what cannot be seen; for what
can be seen is temporary, but what cannot
be seen is eternal."*
2 Corinthians 4:16-18 (NRSV)

The New Normal

Looking back, returning to work was one of the best things
that could have happened to me on my journey towards
recovery. I was met with much love, support and most
of all encouragement from the staff and management. I
did however, find my closest associates paying deliberate
attention to my every move. Their primary concern was
how I felt and whether or not I was up to the mental &
physical challenges of my days, which ultimately proved
not to be so bad.

On several occasions I remember being told that it was hard to believe that I was undergoing chemotherapy because of how beautiful I was becoming. One colleague actually said that whatever was being used in my drug treatment, he wanted some. I smiled, not knowing that these conversations were leading to the title of this book.

One of my most surprising, yet touching conversations during this period was with the person who had hired me into the company, my former supervisor. While at a doctor's appointment, my cell phone rang with him on the other end wanting to inform me that after watching me handle my circumstances with such grace and always talking about prayer, he and his family had returned to church after being away for over 15 years. I guess it's true that you never know who is watching you. Ultimately, he was one of four individuals that reported to me that they either joined or re-joined church after watching me. It is amazing the wonderful and blessed feeling you get knowing that you are in some way responsible for bringing other souls to Christ, while the entire time you're finding your way back to him yourself. Little did anyone know, that during that period of time in my journey, all I could do each morning before starting my day was to say "Precious Lord, take my hand", help me to stand and withstand the day that lay before me.

By now treatment had affected my taste buds, nail color (both fingers and toes), weight, muscles, skin complexion and sleep habits. I could no longer enjoy spicy foods, now taking hot sauce off the table for me. My toothpaste had to change to one developed for sensitivity and free of alcohol. Eight hours of sleep was now mandatory to adequately function daily. But the biggest affect was that I could no longer have my nails done in the same fashion during treatment. My new normal was emerging and taking shape.

It was now November and I was excited because this would be the last month of chemotherapy treatment. It was also the month when we celebrate Thanksgiving, which as an adult had now become my favorite holiday. This is the holiday that holds no expectations for guest, such as gift giving. Plus it leads into the Advent Season, the season of anticipation. So how appropriate was it that my last time to be connected to an IV, containing drugs designed to defeat my cancer, would be scheduled to end two days before Thanksgiving.

As I stated earlier, my brother Lonnie now lived in New Jersey, but phoned me daily to chat. I knew it was his way of checking on me. Many of you may know him as Minister Lonnie Hunter, gospel artist, Stellar Award winner, singer and director. But to me he is my brother whom I have been close to all of my life. I depend on him for his love and support. Don't tell him, but sometimes I even listen to what he tells me to do.

During the summer of 2005 Lonnie informed me that he was asked to produce a gospel music CD to accompany the book "Healed without Scars" written by his pastor, Bishop David G. Evans of Bethany Baptist Church in New Jersey. The book was not about cancer, nevertheless, I felt that the title encompassed exactly how I saw myself coming out of this journey that I now considered my test. Lonnie also told me that the song would highlight his singing abilities, and production of a separate video entitled, "The Cause of My Pain". Once the song was completed it was as though he captured my entire journey, from being misunderstood at work in the beginning to being diagnosed with and treated for Lymphoma. It was as if the Spirit channeled everything I was experiencing through him and produced in song. Both the book and CD were being released in time for celebration of my final treatment.

It is important that we as the recipients of services of the health care industry not get discouraged and shut down, but use our minds and ultimately our mouths in an effort to receive the care desired and deserved.

It was finally here. The last day of treatment and I could hardly contain myself. My oncologist ran tests and met with me after I completed my injection. He informed me that all evidence indicated that the cancer was no more. I began to cry while silently thanking God for never leaving my side. The scripture, Isaiah 43:2 *"When you pass through the waters, I will be with you, and through the rivers, they shall not overwhelm you, when you walk through the fire, you shall not be burned, nor shall the flame scorch you."* (NKJV); now took on a deeper meaning for me. I began to understand Faith in a manner that I had never before. I had moved from just believing in God to believing God.

I could now look at my chemotherapy experience differently. Medical research tells us that the drugs used in chemotherapy are designed to destroy the bad cells that embodied or carried the cancer. I on the other hand, began to see treatment as God's way of eliminating all of the horrible things that I had done to my body over my 47 years of life; thereby permitting my body to recreate itself with his help. I saw myself being granted a second chance, the ability to hit the reset button and become the person that I was originally meant to be.

Now that the doctor confirmed that cancer was no longer invading my body, it was time to have the conversation with him about the subject that had gone unspoken, the sleeping giant in the room; my addiction to the pain medication. I had at this point, been taking vicodin for over six months three to four times daily, and morphine for the first three of those months. So to turn a blind eye to the possibility that an addiction had occurred would be irresponsible. The fact that this was the field that I had worked in for over 10 years, I knew something about addiction. And my goal was to recover on all levels, to include my behavioral and physical health.

When I broached the conversation with the doctor I was surprised by his response. He stated that it was his belief that if a person was in pain, it was appropriate to take pain medication. While that sounds good, more information was needed for me to concur with such a theory. I then asked him what did he see and feel, medically/physically, was the source of my pain since he had now given me a prognosis of being cancer free. He was silent, displaying a look of confusion, so I proceeded with another question. Could it be possible that my body now simulated pain because of its dependence on the pain medication?

He paused for a moment, looked bewildered, then stated that he really had not given the idea much thought. He eventually gathered his thoughts and went on to agree that it was now time for me to slowly discontinue the use of pain medication.

For me, this was yet another confirmation of the importance for patients to play a lead role in their health care; questioning everything even though the answers may not match the desired outcome. I also find it imperative that people look for opportunities to not only be educated by their physician, but to also educate their physicians when necessary. It is important that we as the recipients of services of the health care industry not get discouraged and shut down, but to use our minds and ultimately our mouths in an effort to receive the care desired and deserved.

I left the doctor's office with a mutual understanding that I would slowly decrease my level of pain medication consumption and dosage. I was armed with a new prescription for a different medication and yet, for some reason my spirit led me not to have the prescription filled. All I could see was that I was a professional manager working in an agency in the business of drug and alcohol recovery and that eventually the doctor would no longer prescribe the pain medication for lack of cause, leaving me to search for the drug on the street. I could see the news headlines reading, Cherie Hunter, TASC employee arrested for attempting to purchase illegal drugs. I said to myself, I am not going out like that. So I came up with another plan to rid myself of the drug poisoning my body.

Thanksgiving Day was finally here and as traditions go in our family, I am given the honor of "Thanksgiving Chef". This year I was more than happy to serve in this capacity as my level of gratitude was "off the chain" and I found myself going all out. I prepared a buffet with an array of dishes that the White House would have been proud to serve.

The day was filled with family, friends, love and laughter. But by the end of the day the pain medication had taken its toll. I'm sure that my eyes were beginning to have a glazed over look, as my family began to press me to retire for the night. I finally told them that exhaustion was not the only thing they were observing, but that I was high on pain medications. I knew then that my plan to detox from these drugs needed to happen sooner rather than later.

The overwhelming revelation at this point, notwith-standing the drugs, was that I was now looking at a new normal for myself when it came to sleep requirements, nutrition and medical contact. My new normal meant acknowledging my limitations and embracing my life's reality and all it had to offer.

Releasing the Poison

Thanksgiving was now over. Family and friends were all gone home. Left over food was put away and the house was put back together. There was little evidence of the fun and laughter that had taken place the day before. It was time to turn my thoughts to more serious matters----Detox.

A Special Note: Before going any further, it is important for me to say that self-detoxification is not what I am recommending for people with addictions, as medical monitoring most often is required.

I cleared my schedule the next four days, having already requested time off from work for the upcoming week. I made sure that there was plenty of bottled water both refrigerated and in my bedroom, alerting my sisters as to what I was about to embark upon. At that point I threw the vicodin into the garbage.

I knew if I was to be successful at ridding myself of what I felt was the early stages of pain medication addiction, the process had to begin with prayer. I believed that I would have to follow the directions of Paul in 1 Thessalonians 5:17 to *"Pray continually"* (NIV).

I had no idea of what to expect. I did not know what physical reactions my body would experience, but mentally, I felt that I was strong enough for whatever came my way. Even though I had worked in the field of addiction for over 10 years, I realized that learning and knowing a subject through study, was not quite the same as having to confront it up close and personal. For when I was diagnosed with Lymphoma Cancer and began to research, and study what treatment would, or should I say could be like for me; it still could not fully prepare me for what I experienced.

I realized that everyone's reaction to chemotherapy depended on many different variables. Factors such as how healthy a person is when treatment begins, the various mix of drugs and dosages used in what is called your cocktail designed for your treatment, and the stage at which your cancer is detected. But more than anything, your mindset from beginning and throughout, has an impact --be it positive or negative.

The next 3-4 days challenged me in ways that revealed some inner strengths and resolves that even I didn't know I possessed. I knew that the pain would return, but the extent of pain surprised me. My eyes begin to water and my nose ran. By Day 3 my muscles tightened to the extent that going up and down the stairs became problematic. But I refused to give up or give in. I hit my knees in prayer and told God that I would not let him go until he blessed me or to translate, I was not giving up until my body was drug free. Matthew 7:7-8 says, "ask and it shall be given to you, seek and you will find, knock and the door will be open to you". All I knew was that during this time I was asking until I received an answer; I was seeking to obtain deeper insight and wisdom and I was going to knock or keep pressing my way until the door opened or fell down.

By the end of Day 4 my breakthrough came. The pain receded, my head no longer hurt, the stairs were no longer challenging to navigate and there was an overall difference in my very being. But I knew that if my goal was to ultimately recover on all levels and become the person I was intended to be, I still had to take another step before truly hitting the reset button.

As much as I have heard the statement "It's not about

you", I knew that this period in my life had to be all about me, if ever I intended on helping another human being or myself. So I began to ask God to show me the real me.

I would like to caution you however, before you do this (looking at the real you), know that a high level of pain comes along with this process. Not like the physical pain from a disease or accident, but pain just the same. This is a pain you feel deep down in the recesses of your heart and soul. It's almost like you're Scrooge being transported back to Christmases past, visually encountering all of your past indiscretions and the role you played in them. I ultimately realized that it is our inability to withstand the pain required to make it to the other side of our challenges that stands in the way for most of us reaching the true recovery we desire. Recovery from weight, smoking, drinking, drugs and mostly ourselves, each different in its own right, yet still all challenges that come with this internal pain. For as it says in James 1:22-25, *"Do not merely listen to the word, and so deceive yourselves. Do what it says. Anyone who listens to the word but does not do what it says is like a man who looks at his face in a mirror and after looking at himself goes away and immediately forgets what he looks like, but the man who looks intently into the perfect law that gives freedom and continues to do this not forgetting what he has heard, but doing it — will be blessed in what he does."*

> *"Ask and it shall be given to you, seek and you will find, knock and the door will be open to you."*
>
> **MATTHEW 7:7-8 (NKJV)**

This means that when you're shown who you really are and given a glimpse of the truth that is yours; be it a liar, cheat, back stabber, whatever, you must own it. More importantly, you have to decide what to do with it. And it is in that moment you find yourself at a crossroad.

If you are anything like me, you will cry, you will deny, you will even try to ignore what is being shown to you and attempt to step away from this ever revealing mirror. But as I ultimately and thankfully decided to do, I took off my mask, giving permission for acceptance to come and began the process of forgiveness of myself, and others; allowing my personal transformation and overall recovery to begin.

I was now ready to hit the reset button of my life.

CHAPTER FIVE

Hitting the Reset Button

"Wake up, O sleeper, rise from the dead, and Christ will shine on you" Be very careful then how you live – not as unwise but as wise, making the most of every opportunity."
Ephesians 5: 14-15 NIV

Developing the Process

By now my body, mind and soul had experienced a level of stress that I had never felt before. Needless to say, I was ready to embark on a quest to bring balance back to my life. I knew that to do this required a personal make-over of sorts. So I leaned on the scripture 2Corinthians 4:16-18, *"So we do not lose heart; Even though our outer nature is wasting away, our inner nature is being re-newed day by day. For this slight momentary affliction is preparing us for an eternal weight of glory beyond measure. For we look not at what can be seen, but at what cannot be seen; for what can be seen is temporary, but what cannot be seen is eternal"*(NRSV).

Wanting to live in my own power now, I first looked up the definition of stress, adopting the one that read, "The feeling that's created when we react to particular events.

It's the body's way of rising to a challenge and preparing to meet a tough situation with focus, strength, stamina, and heightened alertness" (The Nemours Foundation). I liked this definition, since it had no suggestion of defeat attached to it. It went on to explain the body's response to stress as being the activation of the nervous system and specific hormones. And lastly it explained how the hypothalamus signals the adrenal glands to produce more of the hormones adrenaline and cortisol and release them into the bloodstream.

In essence, my immune system had been compromised, and some relationships had to be monitored and sometimes put on hold.

This reminded me that human beings function on biology. And since life is the only state of being that biology recognizes, we are created to survive. So it was natural for me to see myself as a survivor rather than a victim.

I continued to study, and learned that there are three critical elements that are the sources of stress: **1) stress of the body, 2) environmental stress; and 3) stress of the mind.** Upon further examination I was able to discern a better description of each element.

STRESS OF THE BODY can be caused by what you eat, the amount of rest you get and also illness or accident. Looking back, I'll admit that I had not eaten as healthy as I could have, unless you count grabbing an energy bar at the gas station while traveling from place to place healthy eating. Neither had I allowed myself proper time for sleep, believing that I could do everything on little or no sleep at all. Then there was the cancer itself which played a major role in my level of stress, as this was a relenting physical opponent demanding attention.

ENVIRONMENTAL STRESS can be caused by where you live, work, music you listen to, who you live with, and relationships. My environmental stress began to take affect when chemotherapy had been decided as my form of treatment. You see, this was a treatment that while intending to heal, also decreases your ability to fight off other things such as colds and flu that could be contracted from others. In essence, my immune system had been compromised, and some relationships had to be monitored and sometimes put on hold.

One of the first things I did prior to treatment, not knowing that I was impacting my environmental stress, was to have all carpets and air vents cleaned at my home. Upon returning to work, I'm sure that I came across as Monk the television sitcom about a detective with an Obsessive Compulsive Disorder(OCD). I disinfected everything around me while not allowing anyone to hug and kiss me, pulling out a "wipe" whenever human contact was made. The antiseptic wipes manufacturer surely found me to be their best customer. But of course, you can't block everything no matter how hard you try.

STRESS IN THE MIND is caused by worries, fears, obsessions, etc. I now can report that being told that your body is being attacked by the disease we call cancer, it can create a certain level of worry and fear. For it is at that moment that you are faced with your own mortality and begin to question your entire life. You fear for your life, while at the same time worrying about how you will withstand the treatment and healing process. And yes, all of these things had manifested within me. I had to fight them off with all my strength now understanding the scripture Ephesians 6:12 *"we do not wrestle against flesh and blood, but against principalities."* Meaning that the ultimate attack comes through the mind, and I had to learn how to put on my full armor for battle.

Being a consummate student in the field of addiction by virtue of my career, I learned a model entitled "Stages of Change". The Stages of Change Model was originally developed in the late 1970's and early 1980's by James Prochaska and Carlo DiClemente at the University of Rhode Island when they were studying how smokers were able to recover from their addiction. The stages of change are: *1) Pre-contemplation* (Not yet acknowledging that there is a problem behavior that needs to be changed), *2) Contemplation* (Acknowledging that there is a problem but not yet ready or sure of wanting to make a change), *3) Preparation/Determination* (Getting ready to change), *4) Action/Willpower* (Changing behavior), *5) Maintenance* (Maintaining the behavior change) and *6) Relapse* (Returning to older behaviors and abandoning the new changes). While supporting, advocating for and agreeing with the Stages of Change model when overcoming addictions and overall change to one's life, I felt that I needed something more immediate to use and/or accompany this process.

Having gone through all that I had, plus me just being

me, I didn't see how these steps alone would assist me with my day to day tolerance of what I had dealt and now dealing with. Furthermore, I would need a process that would support me in achieving the daily peace and stability I needed to exist.

So I developed a process called "Hitting the Reset Button: Bringing Balance Back Into Your Life"; A four-step process that can be applied to your life on a daily and sometimes hourly basis. I began to adjust how I saw things coming into this journey, now viewing challenges as opportunities and stressors as challenges. Ultimately my stressors became opportunities for increased wisdom and self-improvement.

As I continue this chapter I ask that you accept that we all have four areas that govern how we function on a day to day basis. These areas affect us in ways that most often are ignored when we ask ourselves or others, "how are you doing"? The most common response to how one is doing is "OK" without ever examining the four areas that influence an honest answer to how we are doing each day. The areas I am referring to are: **1) mental and emotional, 2) physical, 3) spiritual, and 4) intellectual.**

The area of **MENTAL AND EMOTIONAL** is where fear makes its home. When we examine why we hesitate or avoid facing most challenges in our lives, we would have to admit that fear is what stands in our way. Fear causes us to protect our mental and emotional area, that identifies who we are, with such fervor that even we don't always recognize. We develop a mask that is worn most often subconsciously, for fear that someone will find out what we really feel, the secrets we're keeping or realities that even we have not admitted to. The resistance in facing the fear that is setting up house and moving in all its baggage is what causes us to see ourselves as victims rather than survivors of whatever challenges that may arise in our lives.

It is this area that makes men afraid to cry and women sometimes cry too much. We are taught as young children to put a barrier around this area for fear of it being used against us. To most people, it is believed that if you really examined your mental and emotional state, it may indicate a deficit in your personality. And God forbid we really show how we feel or think. Ultimately we fear living the authentic life we were created to, for fear of what it may or may not mean to the image that we've set up for ourselves. Little do we know, the person being most deceived is ourselves.

The **PHYSICAL** area is the one that we most commonly acknowledge, for here is where we can easily identify if we have a headache, backache, stomach ache, etc. If you are anything like me, you wake up, sit on the side of the bed for about 5-10 minutes looking like an Annie Lee portrait, assessing what parts of the body are working daily or where the stiffness may exist.

This is also the area that most of us embrace or enjoy, because in some ways there is a quick fix---pharmaceuticals. We are in an era where there is a pill for everything. If you don't like pills, there is also a liquid form available to address whatever you think may possibly ail you. Look in your medicine cabinet; can't sleep, take a pill; can't stay awake, take a pill; depressed, take a pill; too excited, take a pill, want to lose weight, take a pill; want to gain weight, take a pill. We now look to pharmaceuticals to relieve, enhance or improve everything about our physical, emotional and mental wellbeing. Self-responsibility has gone out of the window, such as exercise, diet and relaxation.

The physical area is also affected by age, accidents and disease, such as cancer. These are the things that are out of our control. Here is where we deal with genetics, derived from the family we are born into, or we may have had a fall or a car accident; or we may have been subjected to an environment of toxins we were unaware of. No matter how we come to the table, we must inevitably take on the challenge and make the decision of how to respond to it.

This is also where the mental/emotional and physical areas intersect. For it is here that it is imperative that we see ourselves as survivors, gathering the courage and strength that encourages and motivates us to get in the fight. Here is our chance to ask what lessons can be learned and how what we are experiencing will enable us to be a blessing to someone else. Remember, it may be through you that someone else finds the strength to face their challenges.

 It is my belief that we are here to plow and to plant, even if we don't always see the harvest. For when I think back to my mother, though given to me for a short period of my life and none of my adult life, she planted the seeds showing me how to stand in the face of adversity, have faith that the outcome was meant to be, but mostly how to rejoice in whatever state I found myself. She taught her girls how to manage a home, love each other as well as our neighbors and how to continue to press forward no matter the circumstance. Although she was not permitted to see the harvest, her planting and plowing is definitely a large factor in who and whose her family is today.

Now, when we look at the **SPIRITUAL** area, it is important that you understand that this area does not have any implication or depend on any particular religion. The definition of spiritual as found in Wikipedia is: referred to as an ultimate or immaterial reality; an inner path enabling a person to discover the essence of their being; or the "deepest values and meanings by which people live." For it is here that our inner strength and convictions are located.

I'm sure that we have all met someone at one time or another that our impression of them has been, he or she has such a beautiful spirit, even when we really knew nothing about them. This personal assessment of another is because we are all as humans, spiritual beings. And studies now show that most of the population throughout the world acknowledges a higher power no matter the name given to it.

Realized or not, we tap into the spiritual side of ourselves constantly. When we sit down to think, when pondering while looking out of a window, when making decisions, and yes, when we pray. We are asking our inner spirit, to rise up and surface in an effort to help us confront the complexities of daily living.

Some of you may have heard the saying, "the eyes are the windows to the soul". But have you considered the fact that the soul is also where the spirit lives? If so, have you ever looked into someone's eyes and been amazed at the lifelessness seen? Well, it's because they have disconnected from their spirit, their source of light. These are the people we refer to as the walking dead.

It's like buying a plant that requires sunlight to live and flourish, but you place it into a dark room or closet. No matter how you water it or feed it, it still dies. This is because you have cut it off from the source that is meant to sustain it. And just as the plant needs sunlight, humans must always remain connected to their spirit to maintain balance in their day to day lives.

When you begin to purposefully tap into your spiritual area, you learn that this is the area that actually undergirds all other areas. This is where your peace, joy, stability and forgiveness are housed, even when your days seem dark. This is the area that allows for grace in the face of adversity, peace in the storm and love in the midst of conflict.

For if you take a moment to listen to the spirit within, you will find that it sharpens your discernment, permitting you to see past the surface of things. It will prevent you from getting distracted, thus making wrong decisions. It will prevent discouragement, reminding you of the necessity to act. And the spirit will ultimately give you confidence and help you discern the difference between busyness and fruitfulness.

The last area for consideration is our **INTELLECTUAL** side. Here is where our knowledge sets up shop. No matter how much education one has, there will always be some topic, situation or challenge that require continued learning. This is ever so true when it comes to an illness such as cancer. No matter how much you've heard the term, it is still unknown to you. Thankfully, in this age of technology, there is nothing that you can't educate yourself on, thus arming you with information to formulate and ask the right questions of yourself and the professionals assisting you.

This (education) was the one thing that I knew I could control, thus reducing my fear associated with this enemy that had attacked my body. I knew that if I understood the facts, the research and possible expectations associated with lymphoma cancer; the fear and depression attempting to take hold, would diminish.

Most things that we criticize or avoid, are due to our lack of knowledge of the subject. This lack of knowledge is also true when applied to acceptance of other nationalities, cultures, environments, foods and even assignments that we may receive at work. Because we are unwilling or unable to take the time to understand what's behind the differences, it is generally easier to adopt a position of dislike or avoidance. Honestly speaking, it is because we have not examined or accepted who we really are, that places anything different or unknown in contradiction to what we think we know or believe.

Now understanding the four areas that drive us and make up who we are, I ask the question:

If you were a ball consisting of these four areas and one area was removed, how well would you roll?

The Process in Action

I now see that one of the most beneficial things that I did throughout my entire 12 month journey was journaling. It is what has allowed me to look back, examine and ultimately process every step that I took. I realized that in every entry a theme began to emerge building a foundation that highlighted these four major steps, **1) Do a personal check-in, 2) Ask yourself the right questions, 3) Move to meditation/self-examination, and 4) identify the opportunities**; all of which kept me sane, motivated to recover and remain realistic throughout the entire journey. These are the steps I've named "Hitting the Reset Button".

Some days may require that you hit your invisible reset button more than once. It may even be necessary that it is hit hourly, depending on how your day is actually progressing.

Daily throughout my journey I continuously pressed my reset button. When treatment was delivered, press the button; when taking medication, press the button; when attempting to make it through a work day, press the button; and entertaining guests when all I wanted to do was sleep; press, press, press the button.

> *"Some days may require that you hit your invisible reset button more than once. It may even be necessary that it is hit hourly, depending on how your day is actually playing out."*

The four steps in the process are easy and actually something that we do automatically and quickly, most often without knowing it. But if we stop briefly and recognize how we are processing these steps, our outcomes improve.

STEP ONE: DO A PERSONAL CHECK-IN

When examining one's self or what I call a personal check-in, you must assess the following conditions that govern your daily functioning or your response to life's realities by regularly reviewing: *1) Which of the four areas have taken a hit? And 2)Which area can be immedi-*

ately strengthened to support the deficit?

At the beginning of my illness, my physical area had become compromised. This caused me to increase my spiritual area in an effort to support the deficit. As the journey continued and the diagnosis began to be revealed, not only was my physical area compromised, but I felt my mental/emotional area take a hit as well. This caused me to increase my intellectual area by educating myself on the diseases that the tests were revealing. Remember, the mental/emotional area is where fear operates. By becoming an informed patient, my mental/emotional area began to revive itself, relieving the increased pressure on the intellectual area. The more I knew and understood the less fear and anxiety were able to take control, ultimately placing my deficit area back in a more operable and balanced state.

Doing a personal check-in requires you to be honest with yourself to in order to effectively target the specific area that has taken the hit. This will help to identify the unaffected areas that will be needed to pick up the pieces of the area or areas in deficit. This deliberate process of identification is critical. Once you determine the intact areas, you can put them into action, allowing you to have functioning movement throughout the day.

Initially when I received the true diagnosis of Lymphoma Cancer, my mental/emotional area experienced a heavy hit. All of the negative emotions embodied in this area began to surface. Fear, despair, hopelessness and depression all reared their ugly heads simultaneously. Increasing my intellectual and spiritual areas was imperative for proper support. Only through prayer, study and research of the diagnosed health challenge now plaguing my existence, was I able to bring my mental/emotional area back into balance.

I have to admit however, that there were a couple of months that my physical area in some ways, became non-existent, in the support of my daily survival. This does not mean that I ignored how I felt physically, but this was not the area I leaned on for support. If you think about it, there have been times when you have ignored a head ache, a neck pain, or a back pain. But now ask yourself, what helped you to disregard the pain? Whether you know it or not, you increased one of the other areas, as not to submit to the pain.

It should be noted that when one area is decreased and another increased, you must also recognize and do the work required to stabilize the affected area. Remember, all of the areas are needed. This may mean that you change your medical, exercise or nutritional plan to bring back your physical area. You might read and study about your situation or circumstance to improve your mental/emotional and intellectual areas. And without fail, pray, meditate, chant or whatever it is that you do for connection to your spiritual area to ensure its viability.

STEP TWO: ASK YOURSELF THE RIGHT QUESTIONS

When we find ourselves faced with challenging decisions or circumstances, the most crucial step before moving forward, is to ask ourselves the right questions. So often our questions are driven by self-doubt, rumors and most of all fear. Most often we avoid the questions that will truly motivate us to rise to the occasion and allow our inner strengths to be revealed.

It is important that we not only be willing to identify and pinpoint the source of our problems before being able to adequately answer questions, but also address why we are struggling with them. This concept is very important to your healing and recovery, no matter the issue confronted.

In addition to addressing challenging questions that surface in this step, it may help to begin a journaling process. Writing down what comes up when answering questions creates an ongoing opportunity for you to go back and re-examine your thoughts and growth overtime.

The questions included in this step are very soul searching and will require your mental/emotional, spiritual and intellectual areas to be realized and exercised. You should know however, that to get to the heart of the truth, other questions will arise for you as well. These are the questions that I believe will get you started.

1.What do I really know about my circumstance?
Often we look at circumstances in our lives in a fragmented way. For most it is normal human behavior to view situations from only our vantage point, preventing us from considering a view of the entire picture.

One Christmas my father received a wallet as a gift. Before using the wallet, he and my sister sat together to ensure all items in his old wallet were transferred to the new. When they completed the process, my sister disposed of the old wallet and removed the entire garbage bag to the outside receptacle. The next day dad remembered that there had been a $100 dollar bill hidden in his old wallet that had not been transferred to the new. From my father's vantage point, the loss was the fault of my sister, as she was responsible for discarding the wallet. No regard was given to his role in ensuring that all of his personal items were removed from the old wallet before its disposal. From her vantage point, it was his wallet, hidden treasures and all. She felt that once he said toss it, responsibility rested with him; forgetting that she normally double checked his "ok, it's done decisions". So after a lengthy discussion, they agreed to joint responsibility.

For many of our issues and circumstances it requires us to research or engage in a more in-depth study to better understand, or increase our Intellectual area. Sometimes it can be as simple as asking someone else to take a moment to explain details for us to gain a clearer understanding. Just remember, this will require listening on your part, even when what you are hearing causes other emotions to emerge.

Emerging emotions can also serve as a beneficial tool. It is a good thing when we can understand our emotions and what they are communicating about our situations. They can actually serve as a boost towards achieving our potential or living out our purpose.

In many cases, such as health challenges, financial issues and work projects; answers can be found through research via the internet or library. We now live in an era of technology where everything can be researched.

In most instances, more than one resource is available. We must first be open to truly understanding the issue for ourselves, permitting us to fully grasp all possibilities and potential outcomes to make an informed decision before moving forward.

2. Am I Operating from any level of FEAR?
Whether we realize it or not, our decisions are guided by one of two motives; embracing joy or avoiding pain. When the fear of pain outweighs the perceived benefits of joy, we make decisions based in fear.

Fear is a very debilitating emotion. When allowed to go unchecked it can cause paralysis, keeping us from moving forward, thus preventing us from living out our purpose. So many individuals' purpose in life have gone unrealized, not because of their lack of ability, but solely out of fear. If we would only take a moment to examine our inner-being, we would confront our challenges by first asking such soul searching questions as; Is my hesitancy to face or deal with the circumstance being driven by any level of fear, and if so, exactly what am I afraid of? Am I afraid of what this will reveal about me to others or am I afraid to admit or face this for myself? Could it be that I am afraid of failure? Once these questions are effectively dealt with, you can then embrace your challenges as opportunities for growth.

If we were really honest with ourselves, most of our fears are not based in fact or logic, but solely in irrational thought. Whatever the level of fear in your life, it is important that you deal with it honestly in an effort to confront and conquer it. Identifying your fears requires that you ask yourself questions, helping you to have a practical outlook on life, even if your worst fears are realized.

When diagnosed with cancer at age 47, exactly the age of my mother when she lost her battle with cancer, my worst fear had come to pass. Naturally my emotions and automatic reactions were based in my childhood beliefs that cancer meant death stemming from the negative outcome the disease represented for my mother. I had to begin to focus on countering the voice of the enemy with words of truth and begin to ask specific questions to help me launch an attack to recapture a position and drive back my own negative thoughts and misperceptions of the disease.

Ultimately, I had to begin to question anything I believed that proved to be counterproductive to my vision of a successful recovery. This would prove critical and necessary for me to live out my purpose.

3. *Is this my stuff to handle?*
Here is where we ask ourselves whether or not the challenge or circumstance is ours to actually deal with. So often we take on things that are not meant for us to own. This is generally driven by wanting to control what's around us. It can also be used as a diversion away from the things that we really should be focused on.

All of us know someone that can tell everyone else what to do and how to handle their lives or problems, while their own life gets little or no attention. It is said in many circles that children of psychologists are the most unbalanced, preachers children are the most unruly, and teachers' children are the least disciplined regarding education. These unsubstantiated beliefs are based on the assumption that these parents are often; focused on everyone else's mental health, spiritual health and academic achievement. However, such conclusions are only rumor and conjecture and do not represent all children reared by parents of these professions.

In one of Jesus' more famous metaphors he amusingly tells us to stop being so concerned with other people's problems until we've taken care of our own hugely obvious ones. We shouldn't be concerned about the speck or mote in someone else's eye when we're walking around with a plank or a log in our own. Once we've taken out the log, then we can help our brother or sister with their speck.

During my illness this question arose daily for me(Is this my stuff to handle?). Not because I wanted it to, but because my limited strength and stamina caused by the disease forced me to assess things differently. It's amazing how the things you believe to be your responsibility, that only you can do; present themselves in a way that requires someone else to have to deal with when you're forced to retreat. The work that you thought no one else could do but you, the cleaning you thought wouldn't get done without you, the problems you thought would go unaddressed unless you addressed them; you grasp the significance of the fact that life goes on without you.

After coming to grips with the reality that life did not revolve around me, nor would my family or work come to a screeching halt without me there to handle things; I began to restructure or should I say reassess what was important and what was mine to handle. Delegation became a new and active word for me. I also learned to trust that those to whom I'd delegated would rise to the occasion and complete the task. I discovered that when others are empowered, they can often do better than you would have, because they have the time to actually give the task the attention it needs. As my mother used to say, "you need to find your place and get in it". Believe me, there is nothing like the disease of cancer to make you find your place.

4. Am I standing in my power or am I trying to please another?

It has been said that our lives are the sum of our fears. The decisions made by us daily, are what helps us get to where God wants us to be; moving from where we are or experiencing no change at all. It's true that God has given us free will, but if you want to evolve and improve, you must choose not to relinquish your power to misperceptions, fear, painful situations, or people. Remember, nothing can get in your way or prevent your total recovery without your permission. Standing in your power requires you to take responsibility for your decisions or choices.

When we begin to examine or even allow ourselves to address this fourth question we inevitably have to ask, what's best for me? This inquiry begins an exploration and hopefully acceptance of what is keeping us from devoting the time and energy to those things we acknowledge as "what's best". This analysis will motivate us to begin the shift from what we normally do, to doing what is most important in our lives.

For some, the difficulty comes when we begin to sense

the difference between the two. The pain of the gap can be severe. It is then that the feeling of living our lives through a split screen can occur. On the one screen, we feel trapped by demands of other people, as if they are living our lives for us. While on the other screen, we are living our own lives, making the decisions that will ultimately answer the question, What's best for me?

For others, the difficulty may just feel like an unexplainable nagging discomfort. In this instance we are unable to truly reconcile what we are doing, with what we want to do. There are times when we are unable to find joy in what we are doing. And then there are times when we really can't tell the difference.

Too often, we are brought to the realization of this difference in dramatic ways. A family member dies and we are haunted by what could have been, but wasn't; because we were busy striving for success in a dream that wasn't even ours. The company you work for has decided to downsize and your position may be eliminated. Your doctor has given you a diagnosis of cancer with an uncertain prognosis. Your marriage may be threatened by divorce and marriage is all you've known in your adult life. Some circumstances or challenges in our lives such as these, bring us face to face with the awareness that what we are doing with our time and energy have a stark difference from what we believe to be most important in our lives.

It would have been easy for me to conform to the idea of having a port inserted into my chest, granting easier access for the administering of my chemotherapy. But for me, this meant discomfort and an invasion of my body. Where this may have been appropriate for some, (not diminishing anyone's decision or form of treatment); my fundamental belief after much soul searching and asking the right questions, was to utilize my veins if at all possible. This was my way of standing in my own power, which ultimately proved to be a beneficial decision for my recovery.

My choice not to wear a port proved worthy for two reasons. First it eliminated the possibility of infection. Second, it meant I would not have to undergo two additional invasive procedures to insert and later remove the port. And most important to me was that not wearing a port allowed me to feel as though I had a level of power and control of the outcome I desired.

STEP THREE: MOVE TO MEDITATION/SELF EXAMINATION

Here you must take time to reflect, giving permission for your spiritual area to take control. This is where you tap into your inner being, calling upon your higher power to allow your strengths and convictions to emerge and take control. For some they may pray, for others they may chant, and still for others this may simply require a moment of silence. Whichever category you fall within, the step is necessary.

This was probably the step that came up most for me during my journey of recovery. It could be because, when confronted by illness, I experienced a lot of alone time, leaving me to deal with my thoughts, fears, emotions and dreams. Again, the scripture left to me by my mother emerged; *"Trust in the Lord with all your heart, and lean not on your own understanding. In all your ways acknowledge him, and he will direct your path"* Proverbs 3:5 (NIV).

By now you have likely discerned from reading this book, that my higher power is the Lord and Savior Jesus Christ. And during my meditation times a scripture that helped during many of my reset moments was Psalm 109:21-22 that reads; *"Oh God the Lord, for thy name sake: for thy mercy is good, deliver thou me. For I am poor and needy and my heart is wounded within me."* But I also discovered that when we don't know what to say, our spirit knows what we need and will cry out for us.

When you grasp what the spirit is endeavoring to tell you during this moment of meditation, it will be difficult for you to walk away from the direction in which you should travel. Remember, our spirit will grab an opportunity that we almost missed by being blinded to the presence of God in our situation. For it tells us in Galatians 5:16 *"Live by the Spirit"* do not gratify the desires of the flesh.

STEP FOUR: IDENTIFY THE OPPORTUNITIES
Earlier in the book, I discussed the benefits of seeing challenges as opportunities to grow and improve. This final step is where you can look forward to enhancing your own existence, and the existence of others.

Hopefully you have moved fear out of the way and are able to see the situation clearly. If that is the case, you will begin asking yourself such questions as; What can I learn from this challenge? How can this challenge or circumstance improve my life? Who else can benefit from my challenge or circumstance?

If we are honest with ourselves, very little happens in our lives that we did not play a part in. Even being diagnosed with cancer, I had to look back and ask myself, not just what could I have done differently, but what can I do differently moving forward?

I have always been notorious for permitting my weight to yo-yo, depending on quick fixes and weight loss products, when attempting to lose pounds. But upon review of this practice, I began to see commercials and labels for such products with new eyes. I focused on the warnings and small print intended to notify the public under the caption, "this product may cause". And while the language used is limited, almost as if an afterthought, I now clearly hear them when they say such things as "this pill or product may cause lymphoma or may cause some cancers". Needless to say, that if I am to lose weight going forward, I'll have to depend on exercise and my eating habits.

With further scrutiny, looking for opportunities for improvement in this weight loss area, I had to first acknowledge and then accept of my responsibility and ability to make time for exercise. It now occurred to me that not only did I work at a supportive agency, but my schedule was mine to keep. This revelation meant that the excuse of no time for exercise went out the window. Once I admitted my own deficit and inability to see the opportunities, I could purposely design a schedule that included exercise.

Think about it. When we look good, we feel good. When we feel good, we treat others better. And by treating others better, some may begin to ask you how they can do what you are doing. Then not only have you improved your life, the lives of others around you begin to improve.

Once while I was doing a stress workshop for the staff soon after my completion of chemotherapy treatment, I self-disclosed the story of my cancer journey. I expressed how the wigs were now bothering me and that I had a desire to live an authentic life. I then removed the wig that I was wearing in the middle of the workshop. To my surprise, the entire room applauded and told me how beautiful I looked without it. After the workshop, three women approached me to say that they too were battling the enemy cancer. They went on to tell me how my small gesture of taking off my wig freed them to feel better about themselves, giving them the power and permission to choose whether or not to wear a wig.

Throughout my journey, I began to see that when I looked for ways to improve my own life, others were always effected in one way or another. I began to see daily opportunities that presented themselves for me to possibly make a change, improve or just support the existing situation at hand. This was only possible after fear had been removed from the equation.

James Allen, author of the classic book, *As a Man Thinketh*, writes, "The within is ceaselessly becoming the without" meaning "From the state of a man's heart proceed the conditions of his life; his thoughts blossom into deeds, and his deeds bear the fruitage of character and destiny". Only when I confronted the truths that were buried in the answers of these steps, was I able to rise to the occasion and respond effectively to the enemy that had attacked my very being.

Scripture tells us that "Faith without works is dead". This lets us know that we have a part to play in all areas of our lives and that our work, coupled with our faith will sustain us. Our hearts and minds should of course be guarded and protected areas, but not under-utilized.

Once we recognize the power we have in determining our outcomes, we allow our hearts to direct and partner with our minds, and our life's purpose can be realized. We will know what is meant by stepping out on faith, or taking a chance. For if we follow our thought process (and answers received), out to completion by staying the course, it's really not a chance at all.

CHAPTER SIX

Transformation

*"So if anyone is in Christ, there is a new
creation; everything old has passed away;
see, everything has become new".*
2 Corinthians 5:17 (NRSV)

Pregnant with Potential

The year is 2006. I saw it as a new beginning for myself. The cancer was now behind me. Work was exciting again and my family was healthy and happy. Yet something was happening inside of me that I couldn't explain. Daily I experienced a feeling of expectation without knowing what to anticipate. I felt as if an entire new world had opened up for me, though nothing visibly had changed. I hadn't moved to a bigger home. I hadn't received a raise at work. I still drove the same vehicle. But something was different. The sun seemed to shine brighter, and I awoke daily filled with joy. I knew that I couldn't be biologically pregnant, but I could only compare what I was feeling to what I've heard it feels like when you're about to give birth. Difference being that the labor pains had already been experienced and the only thing left to for me do was to push.

This birth was not the natural birth that one thinks of, but birth nonetheless. This birth encapsulated my own delivery. As strange as it may sound, I felt that a new Cherie was coming through the birth canal, yet I did not know what to expect from her. So I lived each day giving it all I had, all while anticipating great things. I remembered a quote by Martin Luther King, Jr. that says "Everyone can be great because everyone can serve, you only need a heart full of grace and a soul generated by love". And at this point in my life, you couldn't find anyone with more grace and love in their hearts than me.

I began the year by returning to the bible classes so abruptly interrupted by my health challenges. Now I could quench my thirst for the study of theology that I talked about in Chapter One. I enrolled in every class that the church had to offer as my schedule permitted. If I wasn't working or in class, I was in a bookstore reading and purchasing books on everything that I thought I needed to understand theology. I bought different types of bibles, dictionaries for bibles, opinions and perspectives, etc. I studied Christian religion as well as Muslim and Judaism. Nothing was off limits for me.

In April I was asked to step forward and take what our Church refers to as the "Deacon Walk". This was a 15 month quest that culminated in being ordained as a Deacon within the United Church of Christ faith. The first 4 months of the walk meant attending class taught by the consummate theologian and my pastor at the time, Rev. Dr. Jeremiah A. Wright. This alone was enough to say yes to the call to serve. But the reality of the call was much bigger than Rev. Wright or me. I saw it as God's way of moving me to my next level of worship, giving and service. So I said yes to the call, wanting to offer myself up to God to use me however he saw fit.

My role at work was also beginning to take on a different look. Although my title or position had not changed within the agency, management for some reason, observed me through a different lens, which also changed how I was utilized in the agency. I was asked to take on the role of trainer and presenter both inside and outside the organization. And for anyone who has known me would wonder, what were they thinking? Surprisingly, I found myself excelling in the role.

Within my family I had never been the sibling requesting to, nor comfortable with being out front, least of all commanding the attention of an entire room of people. Coming from a family of talkers, singers and performers, I was always the one more than happy to relinquish the leading role to someone else. When my sisters and I were asked to sing in our youth, I would be the one a step behind the two of them, as not to bring attention to myself. Even as an adult, when asked to lead a Christmas song under the direction of my brother Lonnie, I requested that the lights be dimmed in an effort to calm my nerves. Now here I was standing before rooms filled with people coming to learn from and hear what I had to say. Talk about hitting the reset button. I found myself emerging as this woman of great passion for working with and helping others, but most of all a woman finally able to overcome one of her fears, emerging as self-confident.

2007 found me continuing my studies to become a Deacon, with the theme for the year being "A God of Restoration". I felt that this theme was chosen just for me. Although it was difficult for me to articulate to others, the feelings swirling through my mind during this period; I'm sure that I exuded happiness and contentment as I reveled in my relationship with God and the feeling of being restored. I believed for the first time, that the dreams I had suppressed for fear of disappointment, could now possibly be realized.

One dream in particular arose through my studies of theology and my new self- confidence. I desired to travel to South Africa to learn about the region. Knowing that Rev. Wright led sojourns to the area, I began to study our weekly bulletin for an announcement. To my dismay, this was the year scheduled for a sojourn to Ghana, not the area of my interest. But somehow this announcement kept coming back to me. So, only as I can, during my prayer and meditation time, I began to bargain with God. I asked that if Ghana be my first visit to the continent Africa, I not go into debt, and be granted the ability to travel with $1,500 dollars spending money. I'm sure God found me to be amusing and reminded me that there is nothing too hard for him.

In preparation for the journey, scheduled to take place in August, I read all the books suggested by Rev. Wright. I scheduled and received all of the required shots for travel to Ghana and applied for an updated passport. No one could believe that I was making such a journey alone, without another family member or friend by my side. But no one had begun to recognize the new me emerging. Just as I had requested, I left home for the airport to travel to Ghana with $1,500 dollars in my purse with all bills and debts current. I laughed to myself and said maybe I should have asked for more. Sometimes I think that God takes moments like this to remind you that he is God and that he can do all things. I took a moment before entering the airport to thank him, asked for travel mercies and just basked in his glory; knowing that it was only through him that I could have come this far.

The trip was all that and more; filled with worship, prayer, fellowship and education. Our main geographic location for our residence in Ghana was the area of Accra; although we traveled to other areas of the region, such as Kumasi and the Cape Coast. Even though there are 47 different languages spoken in Ghana, I was thankful to find English as their official language.

We took part in a funeral service of a tribal chief's son, participated in a wedding on the ocean officiated by Rev. Wright, visited and toured a chief's home, watched authentic Kente cloth being weaved before purchase, walked the route the slaves walked to receive their last bath before crossing the Atlantic, walked the trails through the rain forest, and toured two different slave castles. We were also able to see and go through the "Door of No Return". This was the final door that our forefathers from West Africa walked through before boarding the ships bound for early European colonies controlled by Portugal, Netherlands, Britain and Spain and later the United States. Needless to say, that out of everything experienced, seen or visited, the tour of the slave castles invoked the highest level of emotion in the entire group.

One of the most exciting experiences of the trip for me took place our last night there. A dinner and naming ceremony was hosted in our honor where traditional dancers entertained us and each of us received a new name and were given a certificate verifying the name change. So now my official name in Ghana is Ama since I was born on a Saturday.

While traveling on a bus along the coast, I couldn't help seeing how the locals of the area still fished using nets just as written about in the bible. The more we traveled the region, the more I realized why Ghana needed to be my first visit to the Continent Africa. This had to be the place for me to begin my history lesson as I embarked upon the study of theology. However, my desire to visit South Africa remained.

The year continued more quickly than I expected. It was now December, 2007 and my ordination for Deacon was scheduled to take place the Sunday before Christmas. I was one of seven being ordained. We were given a total of 50 questions to study and prepare for a public quizzing. While some of the questions had short answers, at least 10 of them encompassed 3-4 paragraph answers and we were required to know them all, word for word with no improvising. Needless to say, my study habits and memorization skills were challenged and moved to a level I didn't know was there.

I was now being challenged on all fronts. The hats I wore were many. During the day, Monday thru Friday, I functioned as an Administrator of 8 different programs, responsible for a total of 32 staff. My evenings required attendance and intense participation as part of my walking deacon class study group. Saturdays involved class attendance for ordination preparation, study for ordination and finding time to spend with my father. Sundays represented a full day of Church service, requiring me to attend all three services beginning at 7am and ending at 8pm. I was firing on all cylinders now and found every moment both refreshing and exciting.

With my purpose yet to be revealed, as well as the road God would have me travel to get there; Ordination Sunday found me overwhelmed with anticipation and excitement. Anticipation for what possibilities the role of Deacon held for me. Excitement because not only was my family and extended family expected to attend the service, but my father, who believed in God, just not organized religion; was coming to show his support. As only a father can, he would always set his beliefs and feelings aside to support us in whatever our endeavor, even though now confined to a motorized wheel chair.

Ordination meant standing before the entire congregation of the church, in the midst of Sunday morning service for public examination; and answering questions into a microphone when called upon. When my name was called to come forward, I felt the full emergence of the "new me" fully surface. There I stood, a woman of confidence, pride, courage and dignity; afraid of nothing. It startled me for a moment, but I quickly allowed this new person to take control, pushing the old fearful, unsure woman down into the recesses of my inner being preparing to remove her completely.

I answered all of the questions asked of me without hesitancy, while inside knowing that life as I knew it, was no more. I had answered the call to service and embraced the transformation that was beginning to take place. I realized that the song "He's Preparing Me" was about a lot more than recovery from cancer, but the start of God making me beautiful. Cancer was only the catalyst used to kick-start the process.

My ordination as Deacon ultimately revealed the greatest unseen blessing that I could have ever imagined, authority to administer communion to my father and others. On first Sundays of each month, I found my father's level of excitement increase surrounding my normal Sunday visit. No longer was his joy centered around my presence at dinner and the fact that I always bought him a special treat, but I'd find him prepared for bible study, prayer, singing and mostly prepared for communion. A practice we continued throughout the remainder of his life, bringing us both a lot of joy and subsequently closer to each other and God.

2008 unfolded revealing many unexpected blessings. I was asked to train more often, my health continued to improve, and even my hair had now grown back, but I still wore wigs on occasion. Our church was now under the leadership of a new dynamic and prophetic pastor, Otis Moss III and my outlook on life was nothing short of positive. Then in August, almost a year to the day of my return from Ghana, I received a phone call that I can only call divine favor.

While sitting in my office at work on a Monday morning, the president of the company's executive assistant phoned requesting to connect me with the agency's president at that time (Melody Heaps, President Emeritus). Once on the line, she inquired about my schedule for the next week. Of course I replied that if she needed me, I would clear it. What she said next rendered me speechless. She asked if I would be willing to replace one of our Illinois Senators on a trip to South Africa. I would be accompanying her, representing TASC in a discussion regarding developing a conference on Substance Abuse and Criminal Justice. She went on to say that I would need to be prepared to travel by Friday, just four days later. As most would, she assumed this short notice might be a problem for me given the usual preparations needed to travel internationally. After I caught my breath I responded with a resounding yes, saying that I only needed two days to pack, get my hair and nails done and inform my family.

> *"For I know the plans I have for you declares the Lord, plans to prosper you and not to harm you, plans to give you hope and a future"*
>
> **JEREMIAH 29:11 NIV**

Of course after such a call, I found it very hard to shift my focus back to work. All I could think of was how my dream of visiting South Africa was being fulfilled. I realized that had I not obeyed the spirit a year prior, and accepted the call to visit Ghana, this opportunity to visit South Africa would not have been possible. As I mentioned in Chapter One, I am retired Air Force. So for many years my military ID doubled as my passport. Because the visit to Ghana required me to apply for a passport and get all of my travel documents in order, I was able to respond to the offer to travel to South Africa on such short notice. I never imagined that this trip was in store for me when I obeyed the call the previous year to sojourn to West Africa. I said to God right then, that I would no longer question what he directed me to do, realizing now that only he knows what he has planned for me. Then I remembered the scripture inscribed on my bible cover that reads, *"For I know the plans I have for you declares the Lord, plans to prosper you and not to harm you, plans to give you hope and a future"* Jeremiah 29:11 (NIV)

Again I was packing to board a plane bound for the Continent Africa with one very significant difference. This trip was being paid for, in full, by someone else. From airfare, hotel, car service to expenses, I was making my dream trip to South Africa in style. What a God!

I arrived in Johannesburg, South Africa only to be met by a gentleman holding a sign with my name on it. It was my driver. I tried to act as if I was accustomed to such treatment, but inside I was screaming. He collected my luggage and escorted me through customs to an awaiting extra-large BMW. I asked if he would permit me to sit upfront with him so that he could describe what I would be seeing on the way to my hotel located in Pretoria. He agreed and off we went.

As we approached the Sheridan Hotel in Pretoria, where my accommodations had been arranged, I noticed that it was located directly across the street from what we

would call the White House, the home of the President o
South Africa. The entire grounds were filled with people
all looking towards a stage where someone was speaking
I inquired as to what was going on, only to be informed
that August is Women's Month in South Africa and wha
I was seeing and hearing was Nelson Mandela giving a
speech. I couldn't believe it!

The driver told me that the man, Nelson Mandela, one
of the most inspiring and iconic figures of our age, was
literally speaking steps away from where I stood. I had
followed Mr. Mandela's life since his incarceration on
Robben Island off the shores of Cape Town, to his elec
tion as President of South Africa. I had read his book, "A
Long Walk to Freedom" at least twice by now, but never
dreamed that I would or could ever get close enough to
hear him actually speak.

I rushed through the hotel check-in process, leaving my
luggage with the hotel bellman and ran as fast as my legs
would carry me to get as close as possible to one of the
men I considered a living legend. I was only able to catch
the last few minutes of his speech, but a few minutes
were enough for me. At the end of his speech he spoke
in his native tongue, Xhosa. To say the least, I didn't un
derstand a word, but that didn't matter. Just to hear his
voice and be in his presence was enough. The tone of his
voice literally mesmerized me and I found myself walk
ing back to my hotel oblivious to the thousands of other
people all around me.

I returned to the hotel, contacted our agency's president
letting her know that I had arrived. I had dinner and

rested in preparation for the days ahead. The remainder of the trip was as phenomenal as its beginning. Day two began with a meeting at the South African U.S. Embassy, followed by a tour of Johannesburg's largest drug rehabilitation center. On day three, we took a flight to Cape Town for more meetings. Cape Town was breath taking, from its view of the ocean, to its mountain sides. By day four, I found myself in Cape Town, left to complete our business alone. I couldn't help thinking, where and when did the president of our organization begin to place so much confidence in me, that she would trust me to handle our agency's business internationally.

On day five, I was invited by the Director of Social Development, to visit Parliament and witness the voting on the area's new drug bill. Somehow, I was placed at the same table with the parliamentarians who were actually voting. Needless to say, I was stunned. During tea time, that takes place each morning at 10 am, as tradition warrants, I was approached by the meeting monitor. She proceeded to greet me as an official and instructed me to use the headphones in front of me for translations whenever the speaker(s) spoke in their native tongue. I started to wonder, who did they think I was? I was later informed that I had been listed as visiting on State Department business, which afforded me access to areas not open to the average tourist.

Remembering that August is Women's Month in South Africa, I found myself being treated as royalty. Following my visit to parliament, I received an invitation to a lunch engagement honoring women and hosted by the female

Prime Minister. At the conclusion of the luncheon, a driver picked me up to escort me to do some shopping before the evening events began. Little did I know that the evening event involved entry into the annual African National Congress (ANC) Women's League Conference. This is the same ANC that Nelson Mandela was the president of. I now officially knew that I was dreaming.

Upon entering the ANC Women's Conference, I was given a back pack, hat and tee shirt just as if I were a member. I was greeted with such love and warm embraces that I felt like I too was a member of the ANC. The women danced and sang in a very emotional manner that caught me off guard, and before I knew it, I was dancing and singing along with them. I had no idea what they were singing, as the songs were in their native tongue, but my singing was all about praising God for all that he was doing in my life.

Just as the singing ended, the President of the Congress invited me to the front of the room to say a few words as their sister from the USA. This was the straw that broke me, I began to cry. I walked forward and could only think of something that Martin Luther King once said, "We've come a long way, but we still have a long way to go; so if you can't run, walk, if you can't walk, crawl, but by all means keep moving." I thanked them and wished them much love and success in their endeavor and quickly took my seat.

The evening culminated with an invitation to high tea the next morning, at the home of a wonderful woman (Esther Ramusi) whom everyone calls Aunt Esther. She is the widow of one of the attorneys who had worked with Mandela in designing the constitution now in place in South Africa. By this point, I didn't need a driver, as I was floating on air.

I arrived at her home with my new friend Debbie, who had been such a gracious hostess throughout my visit. Aunt Esther served tea and soup, but mostly we engaged in a very lively conversation. It was here that I learned that Aunt Esther was originally from Chicago and that we knew a lot of the same people. She asked if I had an opportunity to visit Robben Island during my stay. I informed her that I had not. I told her that I was scheduled to leave for Chicago the next day, and that the only tickets available for a tour were after my departure. She immediately picked up the phone, contacted someone, and later told me that a ticket would be waiting for me at the lock for a 10 am tour the next morning. I didn't ask any questions, because I knew that God's fingerprints were all over this trip.

I woke the next morning gazing out at the view from my hotel window that overlooked the famous Table Top Mountain. I said my prayers, packed, had my coffee, dressed in warm cloths, and left for the docks to board the ferry to Robben Island.

I sat on the upper deck of the ferry so that I could enjoy the air during the trip over to the island. While sitting in my seat, I began to reflect over my entire trip and before I knew it tears were falling down my cheeks. Someone once said that life was not about the number of breaths you took, but the moments that took your breath away. And this entire trip had left me breathless. I silently thanked and praised God for all of his blessings, fully knowing that I had done nothing to deserve such an amazing and phenomenal week and that only through his grace and mercies was I given such a gift.

I completed the tour of the island which proved to be the icing on the cake for my trip. I returned back to the hotel for check out and phoned my driver to be taken to the airport for departure. Although the travel time back to Chicago took almost 24 hours, it felt more like 2 hours to me. My dream was ending too quickly and the real world was closing in on me much too fast.

I'm Back

The trip was over, but I returned to my family and my place of employment a different person. I was back to my life; to give TASC, my family, my church, but mostly God all I had. My appreciation for everything around me changed and for the first time I realized that God had not only healed me, but changed my entire life. He was bringing me to my purpose, bringing me back to what and who I was born to be.

It was now time that I remove the final layer of the mask I had been wearing for years. I had moved from having a religion to having a relationship with God for the first time and no longer could any hardship interfere with this relationship I cherished. But I knew that if I were to have a vertical (with God) and horizontal (with humans) relationship, there was something left for me to do.

Before returning to my office, as I had a couple of days of

to regain my footing and shake off any jet lag, I decided to take myself through another process. I remembered asking myself on the flight home, after reviewing in my mind all that had transpired in my life for the past few years: Who am I really? And since I was in no way tired from my excursion, actually energized; I set out to answer this question, taking myself through a personal retreat of a sorts.

To do this, I sat in my living room with a flip chart in front of me, no television, telephone or music; wondering, how I could pull this information from the recesses of my soul, where I was convinced the answers lay. What continued to come up was an evaluation of my morals, values and beliefs. I determined that if I was to ever live an authentic life, one in which God was the center, I had to assess, understand and ultimately reconcile these areas. It is my belief that here is where we as humans battle those internal conflicts that are unrecognizable. In these often hidden areas: our morals, values and beliefs; we rarely, as people ask the question: Are the things in these three areas really mine or were they passed on to me. This means that often the internal conflict waging war inside us is because who we are trying to be was either 1) passed down by our elders or family; 2) cultural beliefs of the community we live in; or 3) cultural perceptions by virtue of our birth.

This does not mean that we are not or should not be somehow shaped by our families, communities or culture. It is however, saying that we must at some point in our lives, become our own individual, trusting that those who love and care for us will do so no matter what; allowing us to

live as authentically as possible, moving to the agape (un
conditional) love God intended. Then I thought abou
what scripture says in Romans 12:2 (NIV), *Do not con
form to the pattern of this world, but be transformed b*
the renewing of your mind. Then you will be able to tes
and approve what God's will is—his good, pleasing anc
perfect will."

So over the next couple of days, I worked through a pro
cess by developing the following form allowing for the as
sessment of where each moral, value and belief of min
really shook out. On several occasions, some items move
from column to column, until the answers to; who am
really, were able to emerge.

Who Am I Really?

Morals/Values/Beliefs	Mine	Given to me	If given, by whom
1.			
2.			
3.			
4.			

I kept my final document, posting it behind my bedroom
door to reference when decision making became difficult
I thought it to be important that I be able to remind myself of my own beliefs and values when doubt managec
to take hold preventing me from moving forward. Each
year I reexamine this document interested in change:
and growth, in an effort to remain authentic in how I live
Hopefully this process will be of assistance to others.

Over the next year, I traveled back to South Africa fou
times to plan the conference scheduled to take place in
October of 2009. However, none of the trips comparec

to my first visit that I can only say was designed and orchestrated by God. The conference was held in Cape Town with participants coming from the entire country of South Africa. And this time I was accompanied by my sister Lonnetta, as I was able to get her to present at the conference as well. Since she is the Executive Director of Great Lakes Addiction Technology Transfer Center located at the University of Illinois at Chicago/Jane Addams College of Social Work, it was a natural and perfect request to solicit her expertise and participation. Plus the conference was scheduled to be held on my birthday, and since my sister is also my best friend, it was great to have her there.

> *When I say that I'm back, I'm not referring to any state of being I once was. I say that I'm back to the person I was born to be, but never was. I'm back to the person I was meant to be, but never lived up to. I'm back to what God intended for me."*

In July of that same year, I also received a promotion at work to Director of External Training and Director of the Center for Criminal Justice at TASC, a position that ultimately catapulted me to national attention as a trainer and presenter. I have now traveled to such places as Puerto Rico, Wyoming, California, the District of Columbia, Arizona and many other places representing Treatment Alternatives for Safe Communities (TASC). I culminated my full time employment with the agency I now call my family, moving into a consultant role. I now head up my brother's company "Hunter Communications Group, Inc." in which I am the Executive Director.

In 2010, Lonnie, seeming to always be the catalyst that

God uses to channel through music exactly where I am in life, also began writing and producing a new CD entitled "I'm Back". I thought, what an appropriate title for the final segment of the book I knew I had to write.

But for me, when I say that I'm Back, I'm not referring to any state of being where I once was. I say that I'm Back to the person I was born to be, but never was. I'm Back to the person I was meant to be, but never lived up to. I'm Back, to what God intended for me. For as the scripture that opens this chapter says; *"So if anyone is in Christ, there is a new creation; everything old has passed away; see everything has become new!"* 2 Corinthians5:17 (NRSV)

So when you hear the words in the song "I'm Back" say, "You gave me another chance, delivered and enhanced; now I can say I'm Back, to give you all I got"; think of me and you will know why I say *"Cancer Made Me Beautiful."*

To God be the Glory for all that he has done.

Closing Prayer

Most Gracious and Loving God, I come before you, a woman moving from battle to victory, because of your many grace and mercies.

Father God, I thank you for the strength to stand firm through all my trials; sickness, fear, addiction, Cancer and through so many other storms and tests that have come through my life. I thank you God for being there when I understood and when I didn't.

I thank you Lord for what you have done, for what you are doing, and for what you will do in and through me; your undeserving child.

Thank you for the deliverance from everything that has been holding me back from being who you have called me to be.

I thank you for your presence right now in every situation, believing and knowing that you in fact, have the battle in the palm of your hand and therefore I know without a doubt that the victory is mine through Christ Jesus who will do exactly what he said he would do.

I Love you, I adore you and I will forever magnify your name.

Amen, Amen, Amen!

The Reset of Recovery at the End of Black

DENISE HUNTER

All the time, all the choices,   All the consequences and the
Colors of our mind, painted with our own brush.
Fear, Rage, Love, Envy, Pain
Blue, Red, Pink, Green,Gray.

The journey through our minds, our lives, our feelings
All leading not to the white light, that would be the end....
But to Black.

Like the children of Israel in the wilderness for 40 years
Not because the promise was not there,
But the faith waivered in the storms.

Once the black cloud comes, the transition through it forces the
colors to surface.
Change comes quickly...
It is the transition that is another color...
a rainbow yet to find.
But ....

If a reset is pushed, the mind renewed, the clouds roll away
the black clouds fade behind us and we see clearly.
No longer do we see through a glass darkly.

At the end of BLACK ..... You Can Come Back.

Seeing the path behind for what it really was
Seeing the present for what it really is
Smiling at your own reflection, knowing you had
enough all along, and now ....

You can move forward toward the promise that was always there
Waiting for your transition into your promise land
The beauty and perfection that is you.

Colors of Ribbons Representing Cancer

Awareness ribbons are pieces of colored ribbons folded into a loop and worn to represent various types of cancer and other causes. They are typically worn to show support for a loved one who has died from or survived cancer. Some ribbon colors represent more than one cause.

LAVENDER
While many other colors stand for particular types of cancer, lavender has been a symbol for general cancer awareness

PINK, BLUES, BROWN AND GOLD
The most widely recognized ribbon is the pink ribbon, which is worn in support of those who have suffered with and/or died from breast cancer. A blue ribbon is worn to support breast cancer in males. Light blue ribbons represent prostate cancer, and dark blue ribbons represent colon cancer. A brown ribbon is also used to represent colon cancer or colorectal cancer. A gold ribbon is worn as support for a cure and as representation for all childhood cancers.

TEAL, ORANGE, YELLOW AND GREEN
Teal represents all gynecological cancers to include ovarian cancer, cervical cancer and uterine cancer. An orange ribbon is worn to represent and support those who have suffered with leukemia. Yellow ribbons are worn to represent bladder cancer, and green ribbons are worn to show support for someone who has suffered from kidney cancer or kidney disease.

PURPLE, PERIWINKLE AND LAVENDER
A purple ribbon is worn to represent pancreatic cancer, testicular cancer or thyroid cancer as well as a representation of all cancer survivors. Periwinkle ribbons are worn to represent stomach cancer or esophageal cancer. A lavender ribbon is worn to represent awareness of all cancers.

GRAY, WHITE AND PEARL

A gray ribbon is worn to represent brain cancer or brain tumors. White ribbons are worn to support someone with bone cancer and might also be worn in place of a pearl ribbon to represent lung cancer.

BLACK, BURGUNDY AND MULTICOLORED

A black ribbon represents a deadly form of skin cancer known as melanoma, and a burgundy ribbon represents myeloma. Multicolored ribbons represent a combination of diseases. A combination of teal and pink is worn to represent hereditary breast cancer or for a combination of breast and gynecological cancers. Black and white ribbons are worn to represent characinoid syndrome cancer. A red and white ribbon represents head and neck cancer when worn, and a combination of pink, teal and purple ribbons are worn to show support for those who have suffered from thyroid cancer .

OTHER COLORS

A number of other colors are used for other types of cancer, although they all also represent other causes. Orange ribbons are used for leukemia and lymphoma awareness along with kidney cancer awareness, while green is also used for kidney cancer. Yellow ribbons are a symbol for bladder cancer, white ribbons are a symbol for bone cancer, and pearl ribbons are a symbol for both lung cancer and mesothelioma.

References

Some Scripture quotations marked NIV are from The Student Study Bible/New International Version copyright 1986, 1992, 1996 by Zondervan Publishing House; Used by permission

Some Scripture quotations marked NIV are from the Life Application Study Bible/New International Version Copyright 1973, 1978, 1984 by International Bible Society, Used by permission

Scripture quotations marked NRSV are from The New Oxford Annotated Bible/New Revised Standard Version Copyright 1973, 1977, 1991, 2001 Oxford University Press, Inc. Used by permission

Wikipedia Foundation, Inc. www.wikipedia.org/wiki/Lymphoma, 2011

Wikipedia Foundation, Inc. www.wikipedia.org/wiki/American-CancerSociety, 2010

'As a Man Thinketh" By James Allen, published 1902. released the 1st of October 2003 as a Project Gutenberg eText edition.

Changing for Good : A revolutionary 6 stage program for overcoming bad habits and moving your life positively forward Prochaska, Norcross & DiClemente (William Morrow and Co. Inc, 1992)

The Nemours Foundation definition of Stress 1995-2011

What Color Ribbons Represent Types of Cancer? | eHow.com http://www.ehow.com/about_5375462_color-ribbons-represent-types-cancer.html#ixzz1ABtPsltB

Cancer Ribbons Color List | eHow.com http://www.ehow.com/list_6870905_cancer-ribbons-color-list.html#ixzz1ABwXY0yX

CREDITS

Lonnetta Albright

Denise Hunter

Funeka Sihlali

Monica Moss

Melody Heaps

Lonnie V. Hunter, III

Jeremy Hunter Wright

Erial Ramsey

Rev. Dr. Jeremiah A. Wright, Jr

Peter Palanca

To purchase the CD "I'm Back"
by Lonnie Hunter and Structure visit:
www.thelonniehuntershow.com

"Hitting the Reset Button" workbook coming soon!

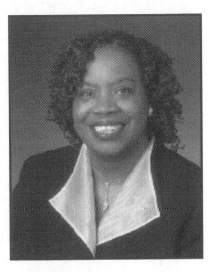

About the Author

Cherie A. Hunter, sister, daughter, deacon, and friend is Executive Director of Hunter Communication Group, Inc. and a five year lymphoma cancer survivor. Sought-after speaker, trainer and conference organizer, with over 25 year' experience in the Human Services field and retired Illinois Air National Guard member. Former Director of External Training for Treatment Alternatives for Safe Communities (TASC) in Illinois and Director of the Center for Criminal Justice for Great Lakes Addiction Technology Transfer Center at TASC. While working in the human services field, she has developed and implemented programs for people living with HIV/AIDS, youth, families and low-income communities, child welfare, juvenile and adult criminal justice, and other social systems. Dedicated to delivering services and meeting the needs of diverse populations, Ms. Hunter is skilled in developing coalitions and working with boards of directors while providing qualified expertise and innovative direction

WWW.HUNTERCOMMUNICATIONSINC.COM
P.O. BOX 1055, MATTESON, IL 60443-9998